vegetarian
pregnancy
& **baby** book

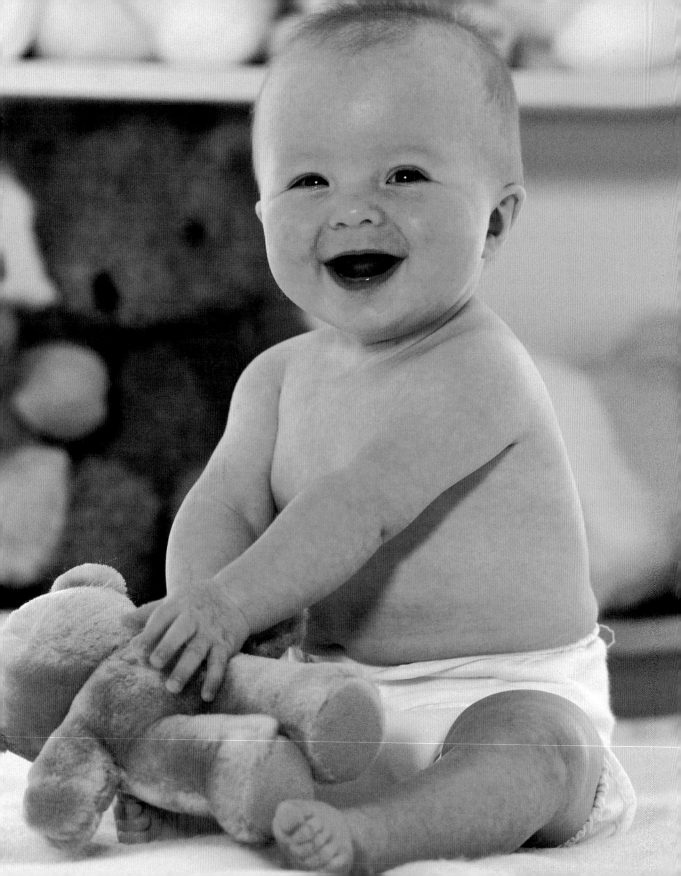

vegetarian
pregnancy
& baby book

amanda grant

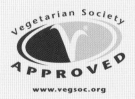

www.vegsoc.org

MITCHELL BEAZLEY

Vegetarian Pregnancy & Baby Book
by Amanda Grant

For Saskia

The *Vegetarian Pregnancy & Baby Book* is meant to be used as a general reference guide and recipe book. While the author believes the information and recipes it contains are beneficial to health, the book is in no way intended to replace medical advice, which you should obtain from a state-registered dietitian, paediatrician, or health visitor. You are therefore urged to consult your health-care professional about specific medical complaints.

First published in Great Britain in 2005 by Mitchell Beazley, an imprint of
Octopus Publishing Group Limited,
2–4 Heron Quays, London E14 4JP.
© Octopus Publishing Group Limited 2005
Text © Amanda Grant 2005

While all reasonable care has been taken during the preparation of this edition, the publisher, editors, and author cannot accept responsibility for any consequences arising from the use thereof or from the information contained therein.

Commissioning Editor: Rebecca Spry
Executive Art Editor: Yasia Williams-Leedham
Project Manager: Vanessa Kendell
Design: Miranda Harvey
Editor: Diona Gregory
Home Economy Assistant: Sibilla Whitehead
Production: Seyhan Essen
Index: John Noble

Typeset in Praxis
Printed and bound by Toppan Printing Company in China

Acknowledgements: Thank you to the paediatric dieticians, health visitors, midwives, and nutritionists for their invaluable contributions to this book, especially to Victoria Morris (paediatric dietician), Tanya Carr (dietitian and consultant nutritionist), and Wendy Robertson RGNRM. Thank you to Sibilla Whitehead, who helped me throughout with research, testing recipes, and lots of support; to Francesca Yorke and William Reavell for scrummy photos; to Miranda Harvey for another beautiful book design; to Becca, with whom I adore working; and Vicki – thank you all so much for all your efforts.

contents

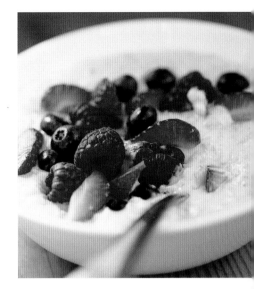

introduction

There are many myths about fertility, pregnancy, and vegetarianism. There is no reason why a vegetarian woman eating a healthy, well-balanced diet should not conceive, give birth, and breastfeed normally. A well-balanced vegetarian diet is extremely healthy for all life stages, including weaning. During this crucial stage of your baby's rapid growth and development it is important to make sure that she eats well to help ensure good overall health and well-being.

I've used the UK Vegetarian Society's definition of a vegetarian as "someone who has a diet which excludes meat, poultry, game, fish, shellfish or crustacea, and any other slaughterhouse by-products, e.g. gelatine or animal fats, with or without the use of eggs and dairy products".

will my fertility be affected by a vegetarian diet?

A common myth is that by omitting meat from your diet you deprive your body of some of the most important nutrients needed to help you conceive. However, all of the essential nutrients needed for healthy fertility can be obtained from a well-balanced vegetarian diet. Any poorly planned diet can result in decreased fertility.

When you start planning for a baby, spend a few months preparing your body for maximum health and vitality, and encourage your partner to do the same. This "pre-conception care" helps you to create the healthiest physical environment for a growing embryo. Ideally, you need to spend at least four months preparing for conception because it takes at least three months for a woman's eggs to mature and become ready for ovulation, and for a man to produce a new batch of sperm. Look at pages 14–35 for a comprehensive guide to a healthy diet, and consider the following guidelines.

specific nutrients Make sure your intake of B vitamins is adequate, in particular B_{12} and folic acid. A supplement of folic acid (400µg) is recommended for all women considering pregnancy and for the first 12 weeks of pregnancy; vitamins D and E are important, as are the minerals zinc, manganese, selenium, and iron. Try to have a good source of protein at every meal.

the pill If you take the contraceptive pill it is a good idea to use an alternative, "natural" form of birth control for at least three months before you start trying to conceive, giving your body the chance to return to a regular menstrual cycle. This is a good indication that you are ovulating normally and that your body is in good reproductive health. The pill can affect levels of some nutrients; in particular, it can inhibit the absorption of zinc, vitamins B_6, B_2, B_{12}, and folic acid, as well as copper and iron. If you have been taking the pill for a long time it is a good idea to be tested for mineral deficiency before you try to conceive.

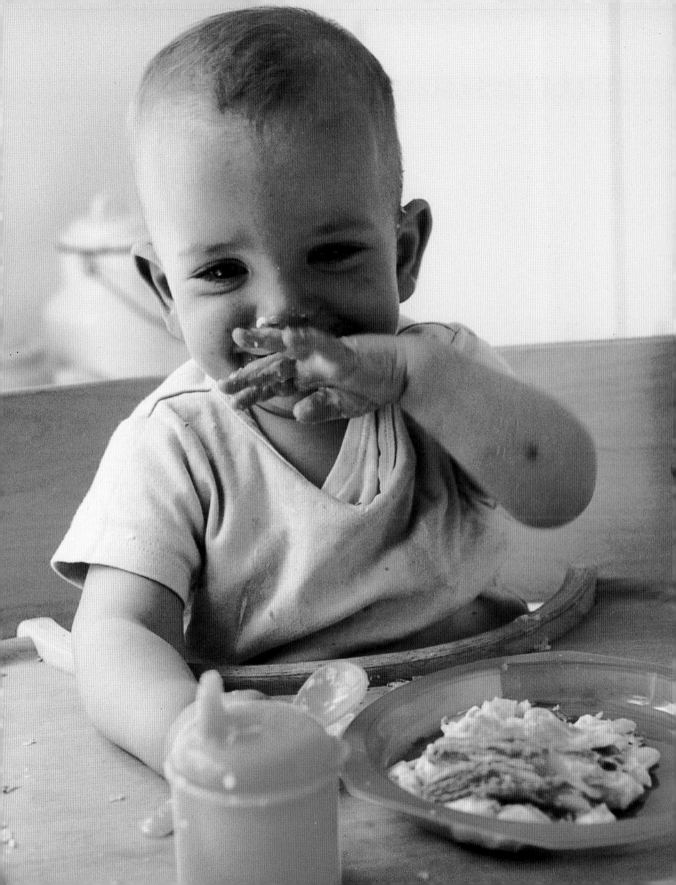

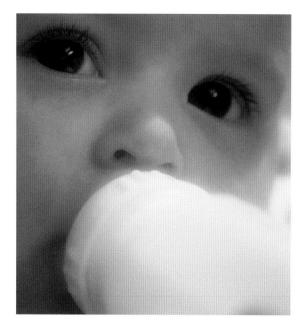

caffeine, alcohol and smoking Ideally you should stop smoking and using any recreational drugs and cut back on alcohol and caffeine, for example tea, coffee, colas, and some energy drinks. Try to drink plenty of water instead.

soy products There is evidence that regularly eating large quantities of soy products (the equivalent of three glasses of soy milk every day for a month) may decrease fertility in some women. Soy is a source of isoflavones, which supply natural phytoestrogen/oestrogen. If you consume enough, you may disrupt your menstrual cycle, making it longer than normal, so you ovulate less over your lifetime and theoretically reduce your fertility. If you eat large quantities of soy products – soy milk, tofu, tempeh, TVP, and soy nuts – it is a good idea to regulate your consumption. Soy sauce does not contain phytoestrogens/oestrogen, so you can continue using this.

weight Being significantly under- or overweight can affect your ability to conceive. Some overweight women stop ovulating and losing even a little weight can be sufficient to increase fertility by stimulating ovulation, improving hormone balance, and making periods more regular. If you are concerned about your weight speak to your family doctor or nutritionist.

organic food Try to eat as much organic produce as you can, even if it is just the basics, such as fruit, vegetables and bread.

vegans Consult your doctor or state-registered dietician before trying to conceive.

will my foetus be affected by a vegetarian diet?

To understand what a healthy, well-balanced vegetarian diet should contain, you need to look at those nutrients you could be missing out on. By not eating meat and fish you are cutting out two major sources of protein. Meat also provides some fat, B vitamins, and minerals – mainly iron, potassium, phosphorus, and zinc. Fish also provides vitamins A, D, and E, some essential omega oils, and the mineral iodine. On a vegan diet, you cut out dairy produce, which is one of the main sources of the mineral calcium. Dairy foods are also good sources of vitamins B_2, D, and B_{12}.

All these nutrients can be provided by vegetarian foods, but you need to eat a wide variety of foods. Use the pie chart as a simple guide (see page 16) and look at the "Foods to eat" section. The recommended quantities of all nutrients for women (and men) are given by the UK's Department of Health as reference nutrient intakes (RNIs). The Government recommends that the RNIs for the following nutrients are increased during pregnancy:

- The RNI for protein for women aged 19–49 years is 45g (1½oz)/day, increasing to 51g (1¾oz) during pregnancy (see pages 21-22). Unborn babies cannot make protein, so it is important that mothers eat enough for both themselves and their foetus.
- The adult RNI for folic acid is 200µg/day; pregnant women need an extra 100µg/day. This is such an important vitamin before and during pregnancy; the UK's Department of Health recommends that "women who are planning to become pregnant should have a daily 400µg folic acid supplement for three months before conceiving, and continue taking it for the first three months of pregnancy" (see page 25).
- The vitamin C RNI for non-pregnant women is 40mg/day; this increases to 50mg/day for pregnant women (1 orange has 97.2mg of vitamin C; 100g (3¾oz) blackcurrants provide 200mg).
- Vitamin A also needs to be increased during pregnancy, from an RNI of 600µg/day for women to 700µg. However, do not be too concerned about eating enough vitamin A-rich foods because the average intake for UK women is 1490µg/day.
- Vitamin D is unusual because sufficient vitamin D is normally obtained from sunlight, so no RNI has been set for dietary sources of vitamin D. However, research indicates that an unborn baby may suffer rather than the mother if she is deficient, so the UK Government recommends an extra 10µg/day during pregnancy. A supplement may be needed to achieve this.

Eating well has other benefits because with all the hormones running round your body during pregnancy you may experience changes in mood, activity levels, and appetite. A balanced diet will help to counteract any difficult swings your body may throw at you.

will my health during pregnancy be affected by a vegetarian diet?

During pregnancy, you may experience one or more of the following conditions: morning sickness, constipation, piles (haemorrhoids), and anaemia. There is no reason why you should suffer from health problems any more than non-vegetarians if you are following a well-balanced and varied vegetarian diet (see page 14-35).

morning sickness This affects many women. It is a feeling of nausea and, in some cases, vomiting, which can happen at any time during the day. It is caused by hormonal and metabolic changes and usually lasts no longer than the first three months. If you go for more than a few days without being able to keep anything down, talk to your family doctor or nutritionist.

To try to relieve the symptoms, eat something plain such as a dry biscuit or cracker or plain toast before getting out of bed in the morning. This helps to keep blood sugar levels steady. Ginger relieves nausea – use fresh root ginger in cooking or drink ginger tea (peppermint and camomile teas are also soothing). Drink lots of water between meals.

If possible, avoid eating foods that can aggravate nausea: high-sugar foods such as chocolate and biscuits, or highly processed and refined foods, because they can be high in additives and preservatives. Similarly, avoid high-fat and fried foods, which can be difficult to digest.

An empty stomach can make nausea worse, so eat frequent small meals or snacks, such as fruit, nuts, and seeds. Eat starchy foods regularly, such as bread and potatoes, because they will help to maintain blood sugar levels and are filling but gentle on the stomach. If you feel too sick to eat, try taking a quick walk before food, as fresh air can stimulate an appetite.

constipation and piles (haemorrhoids) The digestive system is influenced by hormonal changes during pregnancy. The body produces more female hormones than usual to make sure that the pregnancy develops normally. But these also cause the intestine to relax, and it is less able to move food and bodily waste along. Iron supplements can make the problem worse. Coupled with pressure from the baby, this can lead to the development of piles. Another reason why pregnancy makes you more prone to piles – and to bleeding gums – is that the amount of blood circulating in your body increases, causing your veins to dilate. The veins below the level of your uterus are particularly susceptible to becoming varicose (abnormally swollen or dilated) because the uterus places increased pressure on them. To help relieve constipation try to drink lots of water and make sure that your diet is high in fibre.

anaemia Many pregnant women, vegetarian or not, experience anaemia. Symptoms can include pallor, extreme tiredness, and a sore tongue. Anaemia is usually a result of a low iron level, although vitamin B_{12}, folic acid, manganese, and vitamin B_6 deficiencies can contribute.

insomnia Not being able to sleep at night is something that most pregnant women experience at some point, usually during the last 6–8 weeks of their pregnancy. This is hardly surprising – the size of your tummy makes it difficult to get comfortable. You may also be getting up several times to go to the toilet, your baby may be kicking, or you may be woken by cramp. Ideally you will need to make up for lost sleep by napping during the day, but this may not be possible. The following may help:

• Lie on your side with a pillow under your bump and another between your knees.
• Practise relaxation exercises, particularly breathing slowly and deeply, when trying to go to sleep.
• Take a warm but not hot bath before going to bed.
• Have a warm, milky drink before going to bed.
• Have a massage at bedtime.
• Do some gentle exercise such as walking, yoga, or swimming.

heartburn/indigestion Heartburn is common in the later stages of pregnancy and is usually caused by the baby pressing against your stomach. Try to avoid eating large meals by eating smaller, more frequent meals or snacks. Spicy or fatty foods, fizzy drinks, and citrus fruits or juices are best avoided. It may help to sit up straight while eating and to avoid activity just after you have eaten.

weight gain Ideally you need to be a healthy body weight at the start of your pregnancy. If you are underweight, your baby stands a greater risk of having a low birth weight and consequently a higher risk of ill health. If you are overweight, you have more chance of suffering from complications, such as high blood pressure and diabetes.

If you eat a well-balanced vegetarian diet (see page 14-35), you can expect to gain approximately 3.5kg (8lb) in the first 20 weeks of pregnancy. Your weight will then probably continue to increase by about 0.5kg (1lb)/week until the end of the pregnancy. Your total weight gain should be about 12.5kg (27½lb), or about 16–20kg (35–44lb) for twins. If you gain too much weight your blood pressure can increase and you stand a greater risk of becoming obese in the future. It is important, however, not to restrict drastically your food intake because this can adversely affect both your health and that of your growing foetus. If you are worried about your weight see your family doctor or nutritionist. Everyone should exercise to help keep fit and healthy. Adapt your pregnancy exercise routine to suit your base level of fitness. Walking, yoga, or swimming for 20–30 minutes, three times a week, will help digestion and enhance general well-being and fitness in preparation for the delivery. For more information contact the Active Birth Centre (see page 125).

food cravings and aversions It is not uncommon to experience cravings for odd foods and indulging your craving should not do any harm. However, an excessive craving may indicate a mineral deficiency – most commonly iron. If you are worried see your family doctor or nutritionist. Many women also experience strong aversions to particular foods, usually fatty foods, alcohol, tea, and coffee, which are best avoided anyway.

will my diet affect my ability to breastfeed?

Once your baby is born, especially if it is your first, your world may seem to have been turned upside down. The balance of your hormones will be changing and your emotions along with them. You may feel tired and fragile after the birth and that there is no time for anything. It is important to build yourself up after the birth and to make sure that, if you have decided to breastfeed, the milk you provide for you baby is good quality and that there is plenty of it.

All experts agree: breast is best. Breast milk is the perfect food for your baby because it provides all the essential nutrients she needs as well as special proteins, antibodies, and white blood cells, all of which help to protect her against infection, illness, and disease.

There is no evidence that a well-balanced vegetarian diet will affect your ability to breastfeed, or affect your milk's nutritional quality. However, you will need to pay special attention to a few nutrients that need to be increased during lactation (see pages 38/39). Also, make sure that you get as much rest, and drink as much water, as possible.

will my baby's health be affected by being weaned on a vegetarian diet?

There is no reason why your baby should be adversely affected by being weaned on a vegetarian diet as long as her diet is well balanced and varied. The World Health Organisation's (WHO) advice is to breastfeed exclusively until your baby is six months old, then to wean her on to solid foods. However, because you will not be feeding her any meat, poultry, or fish, you need to pay particular attention to protein, calcium, iodine, and vitamins D and B_{12} (see pages 38/39).

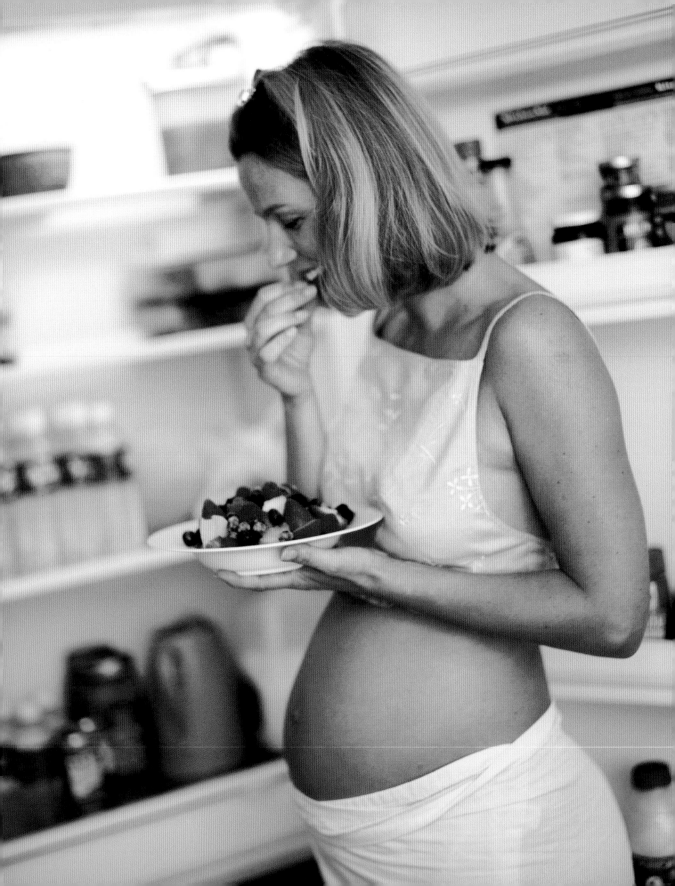

Although pregnancy is a natural process, it needs as much help as you can give it, and eating healthily is the best thing you can do for both you and your baby.

Contrary to popular belief, you don't need to eat a lot more during pregnancy. You may be supporting two people now, but remember that a baby is tiny. It really is quality not quantity that is important: good nutrition is vital for the healthy growth and development of your baby and to keep your body in top condition. Eating well will also have other benefits, particularly on your mood and general well-being: with all the hormones running round your body during pregnancy you may experience changes in mood, activity, and appetite. Keeping your vegetarian diet as balanced as possible will help to counteract any difficult swings your body may throw at you.

While it is important to carefully consider your vegetarian diet during pregnancy, it is never good to become obsessive about it. Eating should always be a relaxed and enjoyable affair.

vegetarian
pregnancy

a vegetarian diet and lifestyle
for the 3 trimesters

During a pregnancy, the 40 weeks are divided into three groups called "trimesters": the first trimester (weeks 1–12); the second trimester (weeks 12–28), and the third trimester (weeks 28–40). A nutritious, balanced diet is essential throughout the 40 weeks. You need to eat a varied diet of good-quality foods for a number of reasons, which include helping you meet your nutritional needs; providing extra nutrition for the growth of your breasts, uterus, and placenta; meeting the needs of the placenta; and laying down stores of nutrients to help your growing foetus and to assist in breastfeeding. Your diet may need to change slightly at each trimester to help you cope with the changing demands of your foetus and your body. If you have any worries about your diet during pregnancy seek advice from your family doctor or state-registered nutritionist.

first trimester
If you find that you are pregnant before you have even had time to think about preconception don't worry. It's not too late to make healthy changes to your diet, but it is important to start as soon as possible. The foetus is most at risk from nutritional imbalances during the first few months of pregnancy because this is the time of most rapid development. Pay particular attention to your intake of protein, iron, calcium, vitamin D, and folic acid. It is advised that you take a 400 microgram (µg) supplement of folic acid for the first 12 weeks of your pregnancy.

Many women feel different: tired and possibly nauseous (see page 9/10). You may begin to feel thirstier than normal, so drink lots of water, and switch from tea and coffee to herbal or fruit teas. There is not usually much increase in appetite at this stage. However, if you feel you need to eat more, choose good-quality foods, and increase your calorie intake by 100 calories a day. Your body will become more efficient at absorbing and using nutrients from food.

second trimester
If you have been feeling queasy or exhausted things may start to improve now. This is the time when many women really begin to "bloom". Your appetite may increase; however, this usually coincides with a decrease in physical activity and metabolic rate, so calorie intake does not have to be increased. Some experts advise that you eat up to 200 calories more a day; others do not feel it is necessary for any increase. Instead concentrate more on eating good-quality foods: healthy snacks such as nuts (see p. 35), and dried and fresh fruit; smoothies and home-made flapjacks; a bowl of nutritious soup for lunch with a wholemeal roll. If you feel a lot more hungry than usual, eat according to your appetite and drink lots of fluid – it's easy to mistake thirst for hunger.

Your body will need more calcium and vitamin D during the last two trimesters to help your baby's bones development. However, your body does become more efficient at utilizing calcium, helping to make it easier for you to consume sufficient amounts. If you include little or no dairy products in your diet, you will need to pay particular attention to this (see pages 26/27).

third trimester

Weight gain will accelerate as your baby grows and your body lays down fat to provide energy. The baby may press on your stomach, reducing your ability to eat average-size meals.

According to the British Nutrition Foundation, you will need around 200 calories extra per day – the equivalent of a couple of pieces of toast topped with a mashed banana. Choose nutrient-dense foods to make up these extra calories. If you are not eating enough good-quality foods during this last trimester and if your fat stores are low, your baby may have a lower birth weight. It is a good idea to increase your iron intake (see page 20). Anaemia, due to iron deficiency, is common in pregnancy whether you are a vegetarian or not. Remember to eat some vitamin C-rich foods at the same time because this vitamin aids iron absorption. If you are concerned about your iron intake talk to your family doctor or nutritionist.

If you are following a vegan diet, finding alternative sources of iron and protein are important (see page 20). Maintaining good levels of calcium without dairy products can be challenging: broccoli, okra, and kale are good vegetable sources. You also need to maintain your vitamin B_{12} level, which is essential for healthy cells – in particular, for cell division and for preventing anaemia. Good vegan sources include fortified soy drinks and Marmite®.

physical activity

Try to stay physically active and to keep fit during pregnancy because this will help your body to change shape, cope with labour, and get back into shape afterwards. Keep up your regular daily physical activity for as long as you feel comfortable, whether it is dancing, sport, or just walking. Remember not to get exhausted and to slow down as your pregnancy progresses or if your doctor advises you to. If in doubt consult your midwife. If you go to pregnancy classes make sure that your teacher knows your stage of pregnancy. Swimming is a wonderful form of exercise because the water will support your increased weight. Try to exercise for 30 minutes a day, but anything is better than nothing.

vegetarian pregnancy
foods to eat

In the UK, the Government gives "balance of good health" advice to the general population. This is often simplified in the form of a pie chart that shows the recommended daily balance of foods to be eaten from each of the five food groups. This advice applies equally to vegetarians, although because of the exclusion of meat and fish from their diets the emphasis obviously is on different foods. The Vegetarian Society in the UK has adapted the Government's "balance of good health" pie chart to suit the vegetarian diet.

"A healthy diet includes plenty of fruit and vegetables and starchy foods, moderate amounts of alternatives to meat and fish, and moderate amounts of dairy produce or alternatives, and small amounts of foods containing fat and sugar." The Vegetarian Society.

It is important to realize that you don't have to adhere strictly to following the "balance of good health" advice every day. If your general diet follows these guidelines you should find it quite easy to eat a well-balanced and healthy vegetarian diet. The chart below shows the proportion of each of the five main food groups that should be eaten in a healthy vegetarian diet.

fruit and vegetables
A great source of many nutrients, in particular, vitamins, minerals, and fibre. Around a third of your daily food intake should be made up of fruits and vegetables. That means eating at least five portions every day: this can include fresh, frozen, juiced, canned, or dried fruit and vegetables.

foods containing fat and sugar
Although some fat is needed in the diet, particularly unsaturated fat from foods such as olive oil or avocados, both fat and sugar should be eaten sparingly. Ideally don't eat these kinds of foods every day, but enjoy them when you do. The recommended number of portions is nought to three daily.

protein-rich foods such as eggs, soy, pulses, nuts, and seeds (alternatives to meat and fish)
The main source of protein for vegetarians. They also provide vitamins and minerals. Aim to have around two or three portions every day, and include a variety of pulses, nuts, seeds, eggs, soy products, and wheat proteins. Do not eat nuts and seeds if there is any family history of allergies.

bread, other cereals, and potatoes
These starchy foods are great sources of carbohydrates, fibre, and protein. They also provide some vitamins and minerals. They should make up around a third of your daily food intake, and that means eating five portions a day. Try to include as many wholemeal or wholegrain versions of these foods as you can, such as brown rice, granary bread, jacket potatoes, and muesli.

milk and dairy products
Excellent sources of calcium, protein, and some vitamins. Aim to have around two or three portions a day. This would include milk, cheese, and yoghurt. If you are avoiding dairy foods choose fortified soy, rice, or oat drinks instead, or ensure other foods high in calcium are included in your diet.

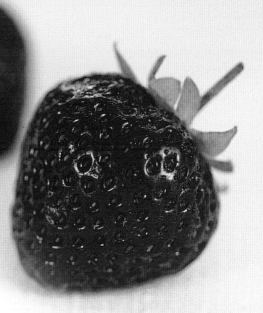

These pages look at the food groups illustrated on the Vegetarian Society's pie chart (see opposite) in more detail, giving you a guide to the sorts of foods found in each group, how much to eat on a daily basis, and the nutrients they provide. You do not have to be too strict about this plan, but if you try to follow the guidelines as much as possible you are likely to achieve a healthy and well-balanced diet.

fruit and vegetables

Fruit and vegetables are a great source of many nutrients, in particular, vitamins, minerals, and fibre. The World Health Organisation recommends eating 400g (14oz) of fruit and vegetables every day. Similarly the UK Department of Health recommends eating five portions of fruit and vegetables every day, each portion being around 80g (2¾oz).

fruit and vegetables: the choice

fresh vegetables

It can be easy to get into a rut and buy the same old veg week in week out, but there are many ways to combat this. Most supermarkets have a large selection, while local farmers' markets, especially in large cities, often have more exotic varieties, such as sweet potatoes, plantain, and okra. Farmers' markets are also good places to buy local, seasonal vegetables. Try joining a vegetable box scheme where fresh, usually organic, local produce will be delivered to your door.

vegetable juices

During pregnancy you may find that your stomach feels full more quickly than usual. Drinking a fresh juice is an easy and delicious way to help make sure that you are getting enough nutrients, and a medium glassful will count as one vegetable portion. Fresh juices are packed with nutrients, especially vitamins and minerals.

dried vegetables, herbs and spices

These are not as common as dried fruits, but there are a few that every vegetarian store cupboard should contain: herbs and spices, porcini mushrooms, sun-dried tomatoes, and peas. Home-made popcorn – from dried corn kernels – makes a healthy snack for the later stages of pregnancy.

frozen and canned vegetables

These can be useful stand-bys. Grabbing some frozen vegetables to throw into a pasta sauce, or to steam and eat with a jacket potato, may help you to eat plenty of vegetables with minimum effort. Generally frozen vegetables are better than canned because they are frozen so soon after picking that their nutrient content is higher; they also tend to keep their flavour and shape better. Good things to have in the freezer include peas, sweetcorn, spinach, and broad beans. Canned tomatoes are great for sauces and stews, and there are lots of vegetables in jars, such as artichokes, peppers, and olives, that are good with bread or pasta for quick and easy meals.

fresh fruit

During pregnancy you may find that your appetite is reduced and you prefer to eat smaller meals than usual with healthy snacks in-between. Eating fresh fruit as a snack helps to keep your energy level up and does not leave you feeling too full. Freezing fresh fruit makes a cooling summer snack – try grapes and chunks of watermelon. Add fruit to cereals or muesli for breakfast, make juices and smoothies, or mix with yoghurt for a quick healthy dessert.

fruit juices

Fruit juices are an easy way for you to eat fresh fruit, especially during the later stages of pregnancy when you may find it slightly more challenging to eat, due to feeling uncomfortably big! If possible, make your own – they will be more beneficial nutritionally because you can drink them straight away before the nutrients start to deplete. Around 150ml (5½fl oz) of fresh juice or fruit smoothie equals one portion.

dried fruit

Ideal for a quick snack providing instant energy, a heaped tablespoon of raisins, currants, or sultanas equals one portion. Banana chips make a good snack and a handful equals one portion, although check the label because some can be very sugary. Dried fruits are high in fibre, particularly prunes, so are great to eat if you are suffering from constipation.

frozen and canned fruit

Frozen fruit, particularly berries and forest fruit, is useful for making smoothies, fools, compotes, and crumbles. Both canned and frozen fruit and vegetables compare quite well nutritionally to their fresh counterparts. This is partly due to the fact that they are canned or frozen very quickly after picking, and also because the processes only cause minimal nutrient loss. Frozen fruit and vegetables, in particular, often have the same nutritional value as fresh fruit and vegetables. If you are choosing canned fruit, be aware of their sugar content and avoid fruit in syrup; look for fruit in natural fruit juices instead. You can buy fruit in jars, usually in the form of compotes, and some can be good – although check the label for sugar and other additives.

fruit and vegetables: nutritional information

vitamins

Vitamins are needed for a variety of functions, including producing energy, balancing hormones, boosting the immune system, and making healthy skin. There are 13 essential vitamins. These can be divided into two groups: fat-soluble (A, D, E, and K) and water-soluble (C and B-complex). Water-soluble vitamins cannot be stored in the body, so foods containing these should be eaten daily. Because water-soluble vitamins can be destroyed by long cooking, especially by boiling, try to eat fresh fruit and vegetables raw or lightly cooked, for example, steamed.

vitamin A has antioxidant and protective properties, which help to prevent damage to cells, particularly those of your foetus. It is also essential for growth, healthy skin and hair, good vision, and healthy tooth enamel. Betacarotene is found in plant foods and converted by the body into vitamin A. Good sources of betacarotene include dark green vegetables and orange-fleshed fruit and vegetables, e.g. spinach, watercress, peppers, carrots, apricots.

B vitamins B-complex vitamins cover a large group of substances, including B_1, B_2, B_3, folic acid, B_5, B_6, biotin, and B_{12}. These vitamins play many roles, including metabolizing food and converting it into energy, assisting in the production of red blood cells, and aiding the development and maintenance of a healthy nervous system. With the exception of B_{12}, all these vitamins can be usually found together in the same foods. Green leafy vegetables, avocados, mushrooms, peppers, tomatoes, potatoes, and beans are all good sources. Fruit sources include passion fruit, dried fruit, melons, whole oranges, and bananas.

B_1 (thiamine) helps the body to convert both protein and carbohydrate into energy. It is also used in brain function and metabolism. Tiredness, weakness, and mood swings are classic symptoms of a B_1 deficiency. Deficiency of this vitamin has also been linked with low birth weights. It is found in tomatoes, courgette, asparagus, mushrooms, peas, lettuce, peppers, cauliflower, and beans.

B_2 (riboflavin) and B_3 (niacin) An increase in protein requirements during pregnancy means an increased need for riboflavin. It is found in mushrooms, watercress, broccoli, pumpkin, and tomatoes. Both riboflavin and niacin work with B_1 (thiamine) to release energy from food. Good sources of niacin include courgettes, squash, cabbage, tomatoes, asparagus, and cauliflower.

B_5 (pantothenic acid) Needed to regulate hormones and cholesterol levels in blood. A deficiency is rare. Found in watercress, tomatoes, strawberries, avocados, dried fruits, and nuts.

B_6 (pyridoxine) Essential for breaking down protein for use in the growth of new body tissues and the production of red blood cells and antibodies. Green vegetables, bananas, and melons are particularly good sources.

folic acid Essential for your baby's healthy development. From conception and during the crucial early weeks, your baby's spinal cord is being formed. If it does not close up properly, the baby will be born with a neural tube defect, such as spina bifida. If the brain and skull do not develop properly, the baby may be severely mentally disabled and unable to survive. Folic acid is also needed to absorb iron. It is found in green leafy vegetables, but it can be a challenge to achieve the recommended daily allowance through diet alone, so it is advisable to take a supplement.

vitamin C Needed for the production of collagen, a protein required for bone structure, cartilage, muscle, and blood vessels. It is also vital for other body functions: helping to turn food into energy, strengthening the immune system, and iron absorption. Vitamin C assists the absorption of iron from plant sources, making it particularly important for vegetarians. Good vegetable sources include spring greens, cabbage, peppers, watercress, potatoes, and peas. Fruit rich in vitamin C include oranges, strawberries, kiwi fruit, grapefruit, blackcurrants, and mangoes.

vitamin K helps with blood clotting and maintaining strong bones. Green leafy vegetables are an excellent source of vitamin K. Some hospitals routinely give vitamin K to new born babies because they do not have an adequate amount at birth.

minerals

Like vitamins, minerals are vital for just about every body process.

calcium Crucial for the formation of bones, skin, and teeth in a foetus, especially in the later stages of pregnancy. It also plays an important role in healthy heart function and blood clotting. Calcium absorption increases during pregnancy so that your baby should get all the calcium she needs. However, if you are a young mum-to-be (under 20), your own bones and teeth may not have finished hardening, so your need will be particularly high.

It is important to include good sources of calcium in your diet when you are pregnant, and to ensure good milk production during breastfeeding. Although dairy products are the primary source of calcium for many vegetarians, green leafy vegetables are also important. Broccoli (especially purple sprouting broccoli), kale, watercress, swede, and parsley are all good sources. Dried fruits, particularly figs, are also rich in calcium. Vitamin D is essential for calcium absorption (see page 27). Some foods can inhibit calcium absorption, particularly alcohol and caffeine. Soy is not naturally high in calcium, but dairy alternatives made from soy are usually fortified with vitamins and minerals, including calcium.

iron Needed during pregnancy for formation of blood and for carrying oxygen in the blood and to prevent anaemia, especially during the later stages. There are two sources of iron in the diet: haem iron from animal protein and non-haem iron from plant sources. Dark green vegetables are an important source of non-haem iron. Spinach (especially raw spinach), watercress, Savoy cabbage, and parsley are among the best sources. Dried fruits, particularly prunes, dates, and apricots, are also good sources of non-haem iron. Iron absorption is increased dramatically if iron-rich foods are eaten with a good source of vitamin C.

magnesium is vital for the release of energy, building strong bones, teeth, and muscles, and regulating body temperature. It also helps the body to absorb other nutrients, particularly calcium and vitamin C. Dried fruit, especially figs, apricots, and raisins are an excellent source of this mineral, which has been closely linked to healthy birth weight. Green leafy vegetables (such as spinach), peas, sweetcorn, courgettes, and parsnips are also good sources.

fibre

Fruit and vegetables are a great source of fibre. Fibre contains no nutrients, but it is essential for healthy digestion and bowel movements, particularly during pregnancy, when constipation can be a problem. Eating enough fibre will also help prevent piles (see page 10).

eggs, soy, pulses, nuts and seeds

These kinds of foods are the main sources of protein for vegetarians. They also provide vitamins and minerals. You should aim to have around two or three portions of these every day. It is very important to eat a mixture of these foods every day to ensure a good mix of amino acids (see page 22).

eggs, soy, pulses, nuts and seeds: the choice

eggs

Eggs are a fantastic food for vegetarians because they are high in protein. The Vegetarian Society strongly recommends that you choose free-range eggs; these should be better quality than battery-produced eggs. Eggs can be cooked in many ways: scrambled, made into omelettes, or boiled and added to salads – the list is almost endless. However, when you are pregnant it is very important you eat only well-cooked eggs. This applies to all kinds of eggs, whether they are hen, duck, quail, or goose. This is because salmonella bacteria are most likely to be passed on via contaminated poultry and eggs. However, the bacteria are destroyed by thorough cooking. Do not dramatically increase the number of eggs (or other dairy products) you eat while you are pregnant because excessive amounts may sensitize your unborn baby to allergies to these foods.

soy

Soy is a naturally healthy plant-protein source, which comes from soybeans, a member of the pulse family (see page 22). Soy is much higher in protein than other pulses – it has a similar protein content to meat, making it an excellent food for vegetarians. The soybean can be made into lots of different things: tofu, tempeh (cultured soybean cake), textured vegetable protein (sponge-like texture, sometimes flavoured like meat), soy milk, miso (fermented condiment), soy margarine, and soy yoghurt. All these products can be used as they are, or instead of meat or dairy products. Tofu is most commonly used instead of meat: it is a popular vegetarian product made by curdling soy milk.

The resulting curd is a firm, cheese-like product, which can be steamed, fried, grilled, or baked. You can also buy silken tofu, which has a creamy texture and is good instead of cream, yoghurt, or cream cheese in puddings such as ice-cream or cheesecake. 140g (5oz) tofu equals one portion.

pulses, nuts and seeds

Beans, peas, and lentils, collectively known as pulses, are the dried seeds of the legume family. They are a great source of protein for vegetarians; however, they do need to be eaten in combination with other cereals to provide a really protein-rich meal. This is easily done – it happens naturally in dishes such as beans on toast, hummus with pitta bread, butter bean paté on toast, muesli with milk, and dahl with rice. Don't think you need to have beans on toast every day. There are lots of pulses, for example, chickpeas and lentils (red, green, brown, and puy). Beans are delicious, I particularly like butter beans, haricot, cannellini, and split peas. It is worth noting some many beans cannot be eaten raw. If you are cooking with dried red kidney beans they must be soaked before they are cooked. Canned kidney beans are fine as they are. Beans and pulses are ideal for dishes such as soups, curries, stews, patés and dips, lentil bakes, bean burgers, and salads.

Nuts and seeds are also good sources of protein; try sunflower, pumpkin, and sesame seeds, including sesame seed paste (tahini). Nuts, including nut oils, can be added to lots of dishes both sweet and savoury – in muesli, in sweet or savoury crumbles, in salads, on top of soups, or as nut butters spread on toast. Seeds and nuts are also an important source of vitamins and minerals, particularly vitamin E. Pregnant women with a family history of allergies should avoid nuts and seeds – see page 35 for more information.

eggs, soy, pulses, nuts and seeds: nutritional information

protein

Protein is needed in every cell in the body to help the body build and repair muscles, tissues, hair, and organs, and to maintain an effective immune and hormonal system. During pregnancy, protein is required not only for the growth of the baby, but also for the growth of other protein-rich tissues, including extra blood cells, the uterus in particular, and the placenta. In short, protein is essential to keep the body working.

Proteins are made up of building blocks called 'amino acids'. There are 25 amino acids. The body can make most of these, but there are eight that it cannot. These eight are called essential amino acids. Essential amino acids must be obtained directly from food. Foods from animal sources, including dairy products and eggs, contain all the "essential" amino acids. Protein from vegetables sources, such as pulses, grains, nuts, and seeds, doesn't contain all the essential amino acids, but if a good combination of those foods is eaten each day, they can meet the body's daily protein needs. The one exception to this rule is soy products. Although soybeans come from a plant, they are very high in protein and contain all the essential amino acids.

amino acids

The recommended daily amount of protein is 51g (1¾oz) during pregnancy. An unborn baby cannot make protein, so if his mother does not eat enough he has to go without. The following excellent-quality protein foods all provide 20g (¾oz) of protein: 40g (1½oz) Cheddar cheese; 250g (9oz) green or brown lentils, boiled in salted water; 400g (14oz) brown rice; 2 medium free-range eggs; 450g (1lb) natural full-fat yogurt; 275g (9½oz) tofu. The main way to make sure that you eat enough protein is to have some in every meal.

vitamins

Egg yolks contain vitamins, particularly vitamin B_{12} – one large egg supplies more than a third of the recommended daily intake of this vitamin – and they are an important source of vitamin D. Tofu contains some B vitamins and vitamin E.

Sesame seeds are a good source of vitamins B_1, B_6, and folic acid. Peanuts are a good source of folic acid. Peanuts and sunflower seeds are also a good source of vitamin B_1, while hazelnuts are a good source of vitamin B_6.

minerals

Egg yolks are high in minerals, such as iron, zinc, and calcium. If calcium sulphate is used in the tofu curdling process, tofu can be a good source of calcium. Tofu also contains phosphorus, iron, and magnesium. Sesame seeds are a good source of phosphorus, calcium, and iron. Brazil nuts are a good source of magnesium, while pine nuts are a good source of zinc. Almonds are a good source of phosphorus.

bread, cereals and potatoes

These kinds of foods should make up around a third of your daily food intake, which means eating at least five portions a day – for example, one portion equals 25g (1oz) dry cereal, a slice of bread, ½ bagel, 50–100g (1¾–3¾oz) cooked cereal, pasta, or rice, or a medium potato. They are the main sources of carbohydrate and fibre in the diet.

bread, cereals and potatoes: the choice

bread

The majority of breads are made from wheat. Wholemeal bread is an excellent source of fibre; granary, wholegrain, and nut and seed breads also provide good amounts of fibre, plus all the nutritional benefits of nuts and seeds. Many white breads are fortified with vitamins and minerals, particularly calcium, but white bread is low in fibre.

If you are allergic to wheat or gluten you could try breads made with different flours: spelt and millet flours are low in gluten. Brown rice flour, potato flour, quinoa flour, cornmeal flour, and buckwheat flour are all gluten-free.

cereals

Wheat, corn, rice, oats, barley, and rye, for example, are cereals. One of the most common ways to incorporate cereals into the diet is with bread, but there are many other staple, carbohydrate-rich foods made from cereals. Pasta is usually made from durum wheat flour. Noodles are made from wheat. Wheat-free noodles are available – for example, soba noodles are made from buckwheat. Couscous is made from semolina, which is in turn made from wheat. Rice is available in many different forms: plain white, perfumed rice such as jasmine rice, brown rice, or unprocessed rice such as wild rice or Camargue red rice.

It is easy to incorporate cereals into your diet. Breakfast can include toast, muffins, muesli, porridge made with rolled oats, or some of the healthier processed cereals – but look out for added salt and sugar in any processed breakfast cereals. Home-popped popcorn makes a great snack, as do plain corn tortilla chips, oat flapjacks, oatcakes, and rice or corn cakes. Try to have some cereals with every meal as they aid digestion and give you energy.

potatoes

Potatoes and sweet potatoes are good sources of carbohydrate and fibre. Make sure you scrub potatoes really well, especially if you are going to eat the skins: all vegetables that have not been thoroughly washed may carry the toxoplasmosis parasite (see page 30).

bread, cereals and potatoes: nutritional information

carbohydrates

Breads, cereals, and potatoes are your main source of carbohydrates. There are two kinds of carbohydrates: simple (sugars) and complex (starches and fibres). They are the body's primary source of energy. All carbohydrate contains sugars, which the body converts into energy. Simple, often refined, carbohydrate, from foods such as sweets, honey, white sugar, and fizzy drinks, is converted into energy and absorbed into the blood straight away – you get a rush of energy, which quickly drops off. Often, you will then feel hungry again.

Complex, usually unrefined, carbohydrate from foods such as wholegrain bread, brown rice, and potatoes (especially jacket potatoes and pulses) is broken down into sugars and released slowly into the blood, giving you a long, steady release of energy. During the last three months of pregnancy most of your extra calories should come from complex carbohydrates.

fibre

Complex carbohydrates are also good sources of fibre. This fibre slows down digestion, so regulating energy release. The UK Department of Health recommends eating 18g (½oz) of fibre a day – that is about two slices of wholemeal bread, a bowl of muesli, one portion of broccoli, and one apple. Unprocessed, wholegrain foods are the best sources of fibre. See page 20 for information on the benefits of fibre.

magnesium

Wholegrain cereal products are all good sources of magnesium. See page 20 for information on the benefits of magnesium.

zinc

Zinc is involved in the process of cell replication, so it is important to have a good supply during the early stages of pregnancy. Low intakes in early pregnancy have been related to growth retardation and lower birth weight. Extra zinc is required during pregnancy, but your body is able to absorb it more efficiently. Good sources for vegetarians include seeds, nuts, and wholegrains.

folic acid

Cereals and bread, particularly those made from wholegrains, provide useful amounts of folic acid and non-haem iron. Fortified breakfast cereals also often contain folic acid, non-haem iron, and vitamins, particularly vitamins B_1, B_2, B_3, B_6, and B_{12}. See page 19 for information on the benefits of folic acid.

milk and dairy products

These foods are excellent sources of calcium. They are also important sources of protein and some vitamins for vegetarians. Milk and other dairy products also contain useful amounts of B_2 (riboflavin) and B_{12}. They should account for around a quarter of your daily diet: two or three portions.

milk and dairy products: the choice

milk and cream

During pregnancy you should use only pasteurized dairy products in cooking because unpasteurized milk may contain harmful bacteria (see page 32). Cream in moderation is fine – it is important to have some dairy fat because it provides vitamin A – but for everyday cooking use natural yogurt or a low-fat fromage frais instead. Pasteurized cows', sheeps', and goats' milk are perfectly safe to eat during your pregnancy.

pasteurized cheese

Some cheeses should be avoided during pregnancy because of the risk of exposure to harmful bacteria (see page 30), but there are many that are safe to eat. The UK's Department of Health says that the following cheeses are safe to eat during pregnancy: hard vegetarian cheeses, such as Cheddar and Parmesan. Pasteurized softer cheeses that do not have any mould or rind are also fine, such as cottage cheese, ricotta, mozzarella (look out for buffalo mozzarella – it has a wonderful flavour), and cream cheese.

Some cheeses contain rennet; an enzyme that is taken from the stomachs of slaughtered calves. A small amount can help to coagulate milk into cheese. If you want to be sure as to whether a cheese contains this or not, check the label. Vegetable rennet will be clearly marked, it may even be called rennin to help to differentiate it from the animal version.

butter and margarine

Whether you choose butter or margarine is ultimately a matter of taste. Butter is much higher in saturated fat than margarine, but it is a more natural food that has a much better flavour and so you may not need to use so much of it. In general, use an oil low in saturated fat, such as olive oil, as much as possible in cooking in place of butter or margarine.

yogurt

Yogurt is full of enzymes, which help to keep the gut healthy. They encourage friendly bacteria and boost the immune system. These enzymes also help the body to digest the proteins from milk, so yogurt is less heavy and taxing on the digestive system than other dairy products. They also help to relieve constipation. Yogurt makes a good alternative to cream in cooking, especially Greek yogurt, although bear in mind that Greek yogurt is much higher in fat than plain natural yogurt. Flavoured yogurts are best avoided in pregnancy because they tend to be high in sugar and artificial additives. Sheeps' and goats' milk yogurts are widely available.

alternatives to dairy produce (soy, rice and oat drinks)

There are a number of products on the market made from soybeans, a member of the pulse family. These include soy protein, tofu, soy milk, miso, tempeh, soy cheese, and soy sauce (see page 21). Look out, too, for rice and oat drinks that can be used to mix with other foods.

milk and dairy products: nutritional information

calcium and vitamin D

Milk and other dairy products provide the best sources of calcium. However, calcium cannot be absorbed efficiently by the body without vitamin D (which the body produces when the skin is exposed to sunlight). Butter contains vitamin D and some dairy products are fortified with vitamin D specifically to help calcium absorption. Eating two or three portions of foods containing calcium will ensure you get enough calcium. Around 600ml (21fl oz) milk will provide your daily recommended intake of calcium. See page 20 for more information.

vitamin A

Full-fat cows' milk and other full-fat dairy products contain vitamin A in the form of retinol (preformed vitamin A). Skimmed or semi-skimmed milk provide almost all the nutrients of full-fat milk, with a fraction of the fat, but fat-soluble vitamin A is lost. So it can be a good idea to have some small amounts of higher fat dairy foods, such as full-fat milk, to ensure that you get some vitamin A. Foods such as butter, Greek yogurt, Cheddar cheese, and cream cheese are excellent sources of vitamin A. All margarines by law in the UK, including soy-based margarines, are fortified with vitamins A and D. See page 19 for more information on vitamin A.

protein

Dairy products and soy-based alternatives provide an important source of protein for vegetarians because they contain all the essential amino acids. See page 22 for more information on protein.

selected foods containing fat and sugar

Although some fat is needed in the diet, particularly unsaturated fat, both fat and sugar should be eaten sparingly when you are pregnant. The recommended number of portions is nought to three daily.

fat and sugar: the choice

fat

Fats provide a source of energy and allow us to utilize fat-soluble vitamins A, D, E, and K. Fats provide essential fatty acids that are vital for a healthy metabolism, the brain and nervous system, the immune system, the cardiovascular system, and our skin – they are necessary to help ensure the healthy development of your baby. There are two kinds of fat: saturated and unsaturated.

saturated fat

Butter, hard cheese, cream, and palm oil are all high in saturated fat, which should be eaten in moderation. A diet containing some dairy products will provide enough saturated fat.

unsaturated fat

There are three kinds of unsaturated fat: monounsaturates, polyunsaturates (including omega-3 and omega-6 fatty acids) and trans fatty acids.

- Monounsaturated fats are found in vegetable oils, such as olive oil and rapeseed oil (canola oil), avocados, nuts, and seeds (do not eat nuts and seeds if there is a family history of allergies).
- Polyunsaturated omega-6 fatty acids are found in olive oil, sunflower oil, corn oil, almonds, and walnuts. Polyunsaturated omega-3 fatty acids are found predominantly in oily fish. For vegetarians the best sources are soy oil and rapeseed (canola) oil, flax or linseeds and their oil, and walnuts and walnut oil. The oils must be unheated (cold-pressed).
- When vegetable oils are processed, or hydrogenated, to convert them into a semi-solid form, such as margarine, some of the unsaturated fats are turned into trans fats. Although these are unsaturated they act like saturated fat in the body and you should limit your consumption of them. Hydrogenated vegetable oils are used widely in processed foods.

fat and sugar: nutritional information

fat

Unlike saturated fat or fat containing trans fatty acids, unsaturated fat should be consumed daily. Omega-3 rich foods are important for vegetarians, and are vital for a baby's brain development.

sugar

Sugar – a carbohydrate – supplies an almost immediate source of energy because the body quickly converts it to glucose. There are two main kinds of sugars: natural sugars found in fruits and vegetables, and refined sugars, such as honey and brown and white sugars, which are found in soft drinks, cakes, biscuits, jams, jellies, and confectionery. Natural sugars are absorbed more slowly by the body because the digestive enzymes have to break down the cell walls first; this prevents rapid changes in blood sugar levels (see page 24–5 – carbohydrates). Sugar that is not used as energy is converted into fat and stored by the body. This is much harder to use for energy than sugar, so it is advisable to restrict your sugar intake, particularly during pregnancy when excess weight can cause added complications. The natural sugar you get from fruit and vegetables is plenty as a source of energy, and you do not need to add refined sugar or honey to your diet.

fluids

You should drink plenty of fluids, particularly as you may find that your thirst increases during pregnancy. Drink lots of water (at least 2 litres a day), diluted fresh fruit juices, milk (soy or cows'), and herb tea. Limit your caffeine (tea, coffee, cola) and alcohol intake (see page 30/31).

vegetarian pregnancy
foods to avoid

The UK Department of Health advises that pregnant women avoid certain foods during pregnancy to help make sure that pregnancy is as safe and enjoyable as possible.

raw and undercooked eggs

Salmonella bacteria are some of the most common causes of food poisoning. They rarely cause damage to an unborn baby because the bacteria do not normally cross the placenta, but it is best to avoid any risk of contamination to avoid any stress to your unborn child. Salmonella bacteria are most likely to be passed on to humans from contaminated eggs. This applies to all types of eggs, whether hen, duck, quail or goose, etc.

Approximately one egg in every 450 in the UK is contaminated with salmonella. It is advisable to choose free-range or organic eggs because their production requires a more stringently controlled system with a higher standard of hygiene than battery-produced eggs. Avoid eating foods that contain raw or partly cooked eggs, such as mousse, home-made mayonnaise, meringues, sorbets, some ice cream, icing and cheesecake. Symptoms of food poisoning include vomiting, diarrhoea, very high temperatures and dehydration. If you have contracted salmonella, drink lots of fluids.

alcohol and caffeine

alcohol

Alcohol affects the absorption of vitamins and minerals, is a factor in raised blood pressure, and can increase your chances of miscarriage. The UK Department of Health advises that if you are trying to get pregnant or if you are pregnant, you should try not to drink more than one or two units of alcohol once or twice a week to minimize the risk to the unborn child, and you should avoid heavy drinking sessions. Ideally, try to drink as little as possible. If you have difficulty in cutting down talk to your family doctor or midwife. One unit equals 300ml (½ pint) (approx four per cent alcohol) beer, lager or cider; one measure of spirits; one small glass of wine.

caffeine

Caffeine is a diuretic: it will make you pass more urine than normal, potentially flushing away vital nutrients. It inhibits the absorption of iron, a vital nutrient for your baby's growth and development. Caffeine is also a stimulant and, like alcohol, it passes through the placenta to the baby. There is concern that caffeine consumption may lead to low birth weight or in extreme cases to miscarriage. It is therefore advisable to limit your caffeine intake. The UK Department of Health recommend an absolute maximum of 300mg a day, but the less the better. Caffeine is more widely used than you might expect. In addition to tea and coffee, caffeine is present in chocolate, colas, other soft drinks – usually 'energy' drinks – and medicines, particularly some headache remedies. For example: 1 cup of instant coffee contains 100mg caffeine; one 'energy' drink contains up to 80mg caffeine; one cup of tea contains 50mg caffeine; one can of cola contains up to 40mg caffeine.

unpasteurized dairy

cheese

Some cheeses can carry the potentially dangerous bacteria called Listeria monocytogenes. Although cases of listeriosis are rare, they can result in premature labour, miscarriage and stillbirth. The symptoms are vomiting, diarrhoea, or abdominal cramps. Avoid all ripened soft and semi-soft cheese such as Camembert and Brie. This includes all pasteurized and unpasteurized soft cheese that have a mould or edible rind. It is also advisable to avoid slightly harder cheeses that do not grate very easily and that are often coated in wax to preserve moisture and extend shelf-life, such as Taleggio and Port Salut. Blue cheeses should also be excluded from your diet.

milk and cream

Avoid all unpasteurized milk (cows', sheeps', or goat's) and any foods containing it. It may contain

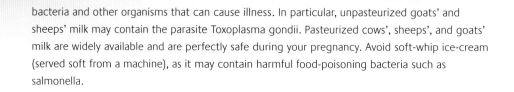

bacteria and other organisms that can cause illness. In particular, unpasteurized goats' and sheeps' milk may contain the parasite Toxoplasma gondii. Pasteurized cows', sheeps', and goats' milk are widely available and are perfectly safe during your pregnancy. Avoid soft-whip ice-cream (served soft from a machine), as it may contain harmful food-poisoning bacteria such as salmonella.

unwashed fruit and vegetables

Toxoplasmosis is a viral infection. It is not usually dangerous and may even go unnoticed in an adult or unborn baby, or just produce flu-like symptoms. However, in rare incidences it has affected the mother and/or her baby. It is believed that three out of 10 people will have been infected by the age of 30. If you have had toxoplasmosis, you will be immune for life – a blood test can identify this. If concerned, ask your family doctor. Contaminated soil is a common source of infection, so wash all fruit and vegetables to remove any soil.

salads

Ready-prepared and packaged salads, available ready washed in bags, may contain listeria bacteria. Also avoid ready-made and dressed salads, such as potato salad and coleslaw. Salad leaves and vegetables that have not been thoroughly washed may carry the toxoplasmosis virus (see opposite). The best option is to buy whole lettuces and tomatoes, etc, preferably organic ones, and wash them thoroughly yourself. The UK Department of Health recommends that all salad ingredients should be washed well in order to remove any soil or dirt.

supplements, drugs and medicines

Not all natural remedies are safe in pregnancy. Make sure that your practitioner is qualified and registered. Contact the Institute of Complementary Medicine in the UK (see page 125) for details of local registered practitioners. Tell your midwife or doctor which remedies you are using. Make sure that your doctor and dentist know you are pregnant before they prescribe any medication.

Illegal drugs can harm your baby. If you are taking illegal drugs, you should talk to your doctor or midwife straight away so he or she can refer you to a maintenance reduction programme. Over-the-counter medicines should be avoided, unless prescribed by your doctor. This includes aspirin, paracetamol, and any medicines that may contain them. Vitamin supplements are unnecessary if you have a balanced diet, and should only be taken on the advice of your health-care professional. Vitamin A supplements should also be avoided as too much can cause damage to the foetus.

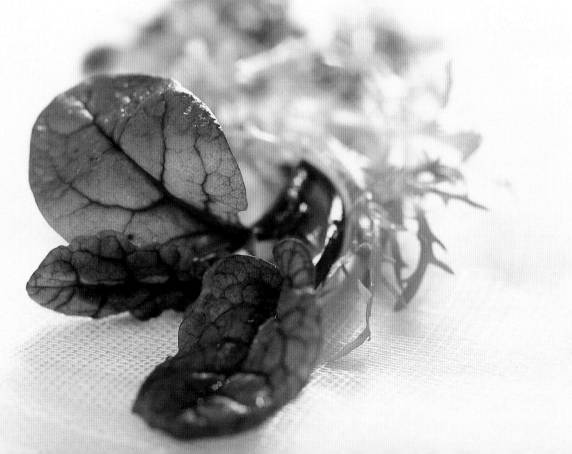

convenience foods, salt and additives

convenience foods

The UK's Department of Health advises that raw or undercooked ready-prepared meals should be avoided during pregnancy due to the risk of listeria. This bacteria has been found in cooked-chilled meals. It also advises that ready-prepared meals can be eaten, but stresses they must be reheated until they are piping hot. The Health Development Agency reinforces this stance.

   The following guidelines can help you store and cook convenience foods properly. Whenever possible, keep chilled convenience foods cool, preferably in an insulated bag or box, during travel and transfer them as soon as possible to the refrigerator.

* Keep your refrigerator temperature between 0°C and 4°C. Always eat foods by their 'best before' date, to reduce the risk that any bacteria that the foods do contain have not multiplied to dangerous levels.
* Follow instructions on reheating the foods carefully. Listeria bacteria are not killed by low temperatures, so thorough reheating is essential. If you are using an oven, allow time for it to warm up. If you are using a microwave, check that you are using the cooking times appropriate to the microwave's power level. Always follow instructions about standing times or stirring because this helps to distribute the heat evenly. Before eating the food, check that the middle is piping hot.

salt

Large quantities of salt aren't good for anyone. Excessive use of salt in cooking can contribute to water retention and bloating, something that may already be a problem in pregnancy. High salt (sodium) intake is closely linked to high blood pressure, a condition that can cause a variety of potentially dangerous complications in pregnancy, and during labour and delivery. Check your salt intake and, as a general rule, salt your food to taste at the table rather than during cooking. Sodium is usually listed in the nutritional information on food labels. Salt is also listed on some foods, but not all. Salt = sodium x 2.5, so if you know how much sodium is in a food you can work out roughly the amount of salt it contains by multiplying the sodium by 2.5 – e.g. if a portion of food contains 1.2g sodium, then it contains about 3g salt.

food additives

Food additives come in the form of preservatives, artificial colourings, flavourings, and sweeteners. For example, more than 4,000 additives, both artificial and natural, are used in the UK. Few additives have any nutritional value, and it has been suggested that many of them have a detrimental effect on our health. At the moment there is particular concern about artificial sweeteners, which do cross the placenta. Although they are said to pose no risk to the foetus they are eliminated very slowly from foetal tissue and so ideally should be avoided during pregnancy. It is far better to sweeten your food with a little unrefined sugar or honey, or use naturally sweet fruit to add sweetness, such as a banana with cereal or in smoothies.

nuts

The UK Department of Health recommends that during pregnancy and breastfeeding you avoid nuts and foods containing them (including groundnut oil) if you or your baby's father, or any of your other children, suffer from any allergic conditions. These include eczema, asthma, hay fever, and any other allergic responses (rashes, itches, and bumps) after eating foods such as peanuts. This should reduce the risk of your baby developing a potentially dangerous allergy to peanuts.

If you can eat nuts, they are a great source of protein, fat, B vitamins, and iron. They make great snacks, but do remember that they are also high in fat and calories, so it is best to avoid eating large quantities of them too often.

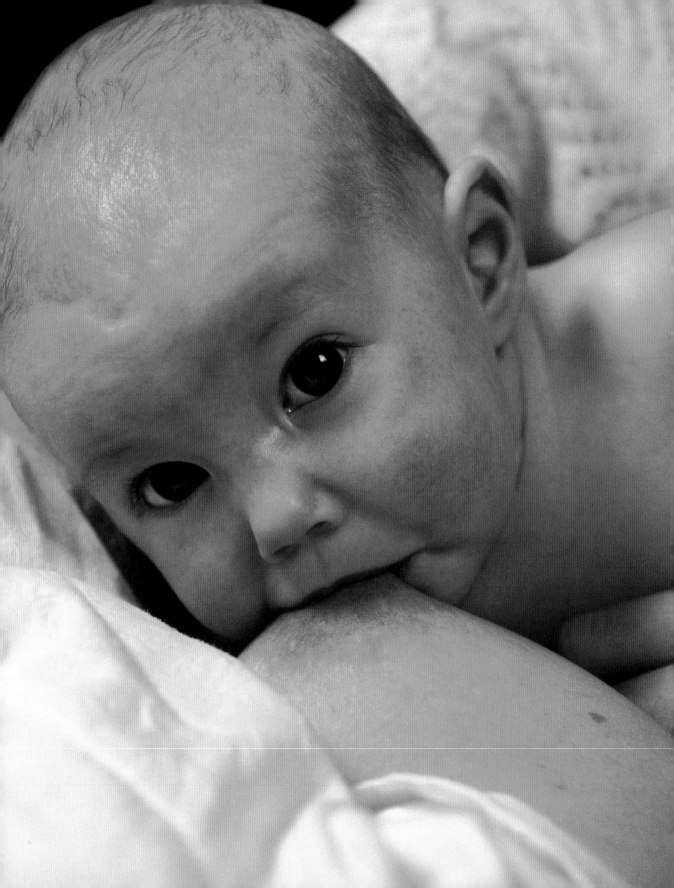

Breast milk is the perfect, and only, food, that your baby needs for her first six months. It contains everything she needs for healthy growth and development. Watery foremilk provides a drink, while the fatty, calorie-rich hindmilk is the main course. Breast milk increases her resistance to many infections and diseases, and lessens her chance of developing allergies. From six months you need to introduce her to solid foods. Your baby will help you to know when she is ready to be weaned by giving you certain signs – for example, she may show more interest in food. When you introduce your baby to solid foods, she will be learning about new flavours and textures, and adapting to eating and swallowing food rather than just drinking fluid. So it is advisable to continue to breastfeed at this stage because her main source of nutrition will be breast milk. However, you will quite quickly be able to move on to feeding your baby a varied vegetarian diet, with your main aim being to feed her the same sort of food that you are eating by the time she is one.

breastfeeding
and weaning

a vegetarian diet
for breastfeeding

The World Health Organisation (WHO) recommends that babies are exclusively breastfed for the first six months, largely because the WHO believes that breast is the best, and only food that your baby needs for healthy growth and development during these formative months.

During breastfeeding, if you are eating a varied and well-balanced vegetarian diet you are also feeding your baby a varied and well-balanced diet because your diet affects both the flavour and nutritional composition of your milk. Eating well while you are breastfeeding is not only nutritionally beneficial to your baby, but it will also help when you introduce her to solid foods during weaning because she should be more prepared for the different flavours of the food. You will benefit from a good diet because it will help to keep your energy levels up and keep you feeling fit and healthy.

You need to eat foods from all the main food groups, providing all of the essential nutrients. In summary, eat plenty of foods rich in starch and fibre, such as bread, cereals, and potatoes; eat a good mixture of five portions of fresh fruit and vegetable a day – it's much easier to do than it may sound; a fruit smoothie could provide you with three portions in one drink! Include milk and dairy produce in moderation and some high-protein foods such as beans, pulses, and tofu. Use fats in your cooking and food, but where possible choose unsaturated fats, such as olive oil and avocados, rather than saturated fats, such as butter. Try to avoid sugary foods or drinks, keep alcohol to a minimum, and particularly avoid them just before a feed. Eat small frequent meals and drink at least 2 litres (3½ pints) of water a day. Do not forget to get plenty of rest, too.

If you manage to achieve the above you are pretty much there. The only other thing to consider is that the UK Department of Health recommends that you increase your intake of a few of the main nutrients, so try to make sure that your diet includes good food sources of these. The recommended quantities of all nutrients for women (and men) are given by the UK's Department of Health as reference nutrient intakes (RNIs). The Government recommends that the RNIs for non-pregnant women for the following nutrients (see pages 12–29: foods to eat) are increased during breastfeeding:

- The protein RNI of 45g (1½oz)/day for women aged 19–49 years increases to 56g (2oz).
- The vitamin C RNI of 40mg/day increases to 70mg.
- The vitamin A RNI of 600µg/day increases to 950µg.
- The vitamin B_2 RNI of 1.1mg/day increases to 1.6mg.

- The vitamin B_{12} RNI for non-pregnant and pregnant women is 1.5µg/day, which is a very small amount. The average intake for women in the UK is 5.4µg/day, which suggests that few women are likely to be deficient. The RNI for lactating women is 2.0µg/day.
- Lactating women need additional vitamin B_3 to maintain adequate levels in breast milk.
- Because sufficient vitamin D is obtained from sunlight, no RNI has been set for dietary sources of vitamin D for non-pregnant women. However, lower levels of vitamin D are found on the foetal side of the placenta than the maternal side. To avoid low levels in your baby, it is recommended that pregnant and breastfeeding women should have a minimum of 10µg/day of dietary vitamin D. A supplement may be needed to achieve this amount, but speak to your family doctor or nutritionist first.
- The calcium RNI of 700mg/day increases to 550mg.
- The magnesium RNI of 270mg/day increases to 320mg.
- The dietary requirement for zinc for non-pregnant women is 7mg/day; this needs to be increased during breastfeeding by an extra 6mg/day for the first four months, then just 2.5mg/day from four months onward.
- The copper RNI of 1.2mg/dayincreases to 1.5mg.
- The selenium RNI of 60µg/day increases to 75µg/day.

Breastfeeding is an energy-demanding activity because breast milk has to contain enough energy to supply the needs of your growing baby. Even taking into account the fact that your body fat, stored during pregnancy, is used to supply some of that energy, you'll need additional energy intake over and above your pre-pregnancy intake during breastfeeding.

Your baby's immature immune system is much more likely to react favourably to breast milk than formula (most brands are based on cows' milk protein). This is particularly true in families with a strong history of food allergies or allergies such as eczema or asthma. If, however, while you are breastfeeding your baby, you notice any symptoms such as diarrhoea, vomiting, or rashes, or if you have a family history of allergies to food, speak to your family doctor, paediatrician, or nutritionist, who may recommend removing certain foods from your diet.

the role
of milk

Breast milk or formula should be the main drink given during the first year. Fresh cows', goats', or sheeps' milk, and soy drinks (other than soy infant formula milk) should not be given as a drink to babies under the age of 12 months.

water Breastfed babies do not need water, unlike those fed on formula, because breast milk provides your baby with watery milk at the beginning of a feed. However, it is still advisable to get them used to drinking water. Cooled, boiled tap water should be offered once you start weaning. Check labels when using bottled water because many natural mineral waters have a high mineral content unsuitable for babies. It should also be boiled.

fruit juice Only give after six months, at meal times once you are weaning. It should be very dilute and in a feeding cup.

breast milk The perfect food for your baby. It is a complete food that provides all the nutrients, energy, and liquid that she needs during her first six months. The World Health Organisation (WHO) and the UK Department of Health recommend exclusive breastfeeding up to the age of six months and breastfeeding at least up to the age of 12 months, if possible, alongside weaning. Breast milk is still recommended as the main nutritional source once weaning begins until your baby is eating a varied diet. The only two main nutrients deficient in breast milk are iron – but babies are born with a store of iron which lasts for at least six months – and vitamin D, so take your baby outside for at least 30 minutes each day, so she can make this vitamin from sunlight.

alternatives to breast milk

It is a good idea to consult your family doctor, midwife, health visitor, nurse, nutritionist, or the National Childbirth Trust for more information about breast milk alternatives before making a decision about which to use.

infant formula milks provide a sole source of nourishment for a baby's first six months. They are more likely to trigger an allergic reaction than breast milk because they are based on cows' milk protein. If you have a family history of allergies, seek advice before you start formula milk feeding.

organic infant formula milks Made with organic ingredients and guaranteed to be GM free.

specialized infant formula milks Hydrolysed protein infant formula can be prescribed by your family doctor if your baby has an allergy to cows' milk. These formulas can be nutritionally better than soy-based milks.

soy infant formula or soy milks There is no particular health benefit associated with, nor any unique clinical condition that requires, the consumption of soy-based infant formula by healthy infants.

follow-on milks These are not intended as a sole source of nutrition, but part of a mixed diet.

how to wean
on a vegetarian diet

The World Health Organisation and the UK Department of Health recommend that weaning should begin at six months for all healthy infants. There appears to be no health advantage in introducing solids before six months, but all babies are different and if you have any concerns do seek advice from your health visitor or family doctor. Starting weaning too early can cause allergic reactions. The UK Department of Health recommends that four months (17 weeks) is the absolute earliest that solids should be introduced.

Weaning gradually introduces your baby to 'solid' food for nutritional and social reasons. Breast milk or formula milk is a dilute food, containing a high percentage of water, so as your baby grows milk alone will not satisfy her. Look out for these signs to see if she is ready to be weaned: she is six months old; she can sit up and hold herself; she has lost her tongue thrust reflex, which pushes things out of her mouth; she wants to chew on things; she still seems to be hungry after a milk feed, and demands feeds more often. If her appetite seems to be increasing quite quickly much before she reaches six months, this may indicate a growth spurt, so increase her breast milk intake before introducing solid foods. However, all babies are individual, talk to your health visitor if you are concerned.

Solid foods are more concentrated in terms of nutrients than breast milk, so even tiny amounts will help to satisfy your baby's increasing nutritional needs. A single food, such as mashed carrot, may be high in certain nutrients, but low in others, so it is important that your baby has a varied and balanced diet of solid foods to ensure healthy development. This is particularly true for vegetarian babies, who get many nutrients from plant sources, which often need to be eaten in combination to get maximum nutritional benefits

Breast milk continues to be the primary source of nutrition for your baby at six months, although some of your baby's stores of minerals, especially iron and zinc, are depleted and adequate sources are needed in her diet. Help your baby adjust to weaning by starting her off with baby rice for a couple of days, then progress to single vegetable purées and then fruit purées for the first couple of weeks. You can then quite quickly introduce slightly thicker purées of mixed fruit or vegetables.

Your baby may prefer to feed herself once you have been weaning for a while. If your baby is ready to move a piece of food from hand to mouth, she is probably ready to bite and chew food (with or without teeth). Never leave your baby unattended when she is eating.

As your baby's digestive system gets used to solids you can introduce more protein, carbohydrate, and energy-rich foods. At 10–12 months she can, with a few exceptions, eat the same foods as you – just mashed up as necessary.

weaning
foods to feed your baby

fruit and vegetables

When you start to wean, the best food to begin with is baby rice, followed a couple of days later with selected puréed vegetables. These are the most easily digested foods for your baby's developing digestive system and the ones least likely to cause an allergy. All fruit and vegetables should be washed and peeled. Always remove the core, pips, and any discoloured areas. Make sure fruit and vegetables are ripe or they might be indigestible, or need extra cooking, which will diminish their nutritional content. Use baby rice and water to adjust the purée's consistency or to soften flavours that may be too strong.

Single fruit or vegetable purées are a great way to introduce your baby to a variety of tastes, and textures. The less strongly flavoured vegetables are the best to start: avocados are easily digested and can be given raw; peas, carrots, parsnips, and sweet potatoes are also good, although root vegetables are high in fibre and may need to be thinned with a little water or baby rice to make them more digestible; broccoli, cauliflower, courgettes, and asparagus are also excellent. Avoid citrus fruits.

Give vegetable purées at the start of weaning to get your baby used to savoury flavours. Breast milk is naturally sweet, so babies often prefer sweet foods, and then introducing vegetables after fruit can be problematic. All fruit, excluding bananas, should be cooked when you start weaning. Good first fruit include pears, ripe bananas and mangoes.

As your baby gets more used to solid food, you can make the purées thicker, then start to mash the vegetables. After around six weeks of weaning you can give your baby more raw fruit and vegetables, so long as they are soft and there is no risk of choking, but they are not as easily digested as cooked food, so introduce them gradually.

Fruit and vegetables contain a concentrated supply of vitamins, particularly vitamins C and A, minerals, trace elements, and beneficial enzymes, which can be absorbed into your baby's system. Enzymes are particularly important because they are essential to every stage of metabolism. Vitamins are needed for a variety of functions. Vitamin C is an antioxidant vitamin well known for helping to prevent life-threatening diseases and boosting the immune system. Vitamin C is needed for growth and healthy body tissue and is important in the healing of wounds. It also helps with the absorption of iron and, probably, zinc. Vitamin C is present in breast milk and formula, but once weaning begins your baby can get vitamin C from fruit and vegetables: the best sources for her are mangoes, papayas, raspberries, peaches, broccoli, spinach, potatoes and peas.

Once weaning is under way you should aim to give two portions of fruit and vegetables a day, increasing to three to four portions after nine months.

Betacarotene is found in plant food and converted by the body into vitamin A. Vitamin A is needed for growth, development, healthy skin and hair, and good vision. Only a limited number of foods, other than milk, contain vitamin A: ask your doctor if your baby needs vitamin drops. Good sources of betacarotene include orange-fleshed fruit and vegetables (citrus fruits are not suitable for babies under seven months), leeks, courgettes, and broccoli.

Green leafy vegetables are important sources of folic acid. This is crucial for your baby's healthy development, as it helps the body to absorb iron needed for healthy blood cells and preventing anaemia. After seven months, good sources of folic acid include pulses and finely ground nuts (do not give nuts if there is a family history of food allergies).

Fruits and vegetables are an important source of minerals, particularly iron. Babies are born with a natural store of iron, but by six months this will be depleted. The level of iron in breast milk is low, but because about 50 per cent of it is absorbed – a high absorption rate for iron – this makes an important contribution for your breastfed baby during early weaning. Many formula milks are fortified with iron. Nevertheless, once weaning is under way make sure your baby's diet has good sources of iron. The best vegetable sources suitable for weaning babies of seven months and older include beans, tofu, a little puréed dried fruits (particularly unsulphured apricots), and green vegetables. Avoid giving high-fibre cereals because they inhibit iron absorption. Vitamin C aids iron absorption, so it's a good idea to give foods containing iron and foods containing vitamin C at the same meal – for example, mango and dried apricot purée, or potato and spinach purée.

eggs, soy, pulses, nuts and seeds

These foods will be your baby's main sources of protein after weaning. During her first six to eight months she will get all of her protein requirements from breast milk, but as she grows she will need a more concentrated source from solid food. As babies grow so rapidly, they need more protein than adults compared to their body weight, so protein intake is vital during weaning. Protein consists of building blocks called 'amino acids'. There are two types of amino acids: essential and non-essential (see page 22). Foods that are high in protein are harder for your baby's digestive system to cope with, so they should be introduced gradually. Give her a month or so on fruits and vegetables before introducing protein-rich foods and don't introduce protein-rich foods until your baby is seven months. At first, mix them with an easily digestible food, such as a puréed vegetable (such as carrot and lentil purée). When your baby is used to protein-rich food, aim to give her at least two portions a day. From seven months she could have smooth nut butter on bread (if there is no family history of nut allergies) or puréed butter beans and leeks.

Eggs can be given after seven months, but they should always be well cooked. Small amounts of full-fat dairy products or calcium-enriched soy dairy alternatives can also be given after seven months, as excellent sources of protein. They are best mixed with other foods to make them easier to digest. Eggs, milk, and dairy products are a good source of vitamin B_{12}.

Soy products should not be the sole or major source of protein for weaning because they are relatively low in calories, but high in fibre – they may satisfy your baby's appetite before she has taken in enough energy. Some textured vegetable protein (TVP) can be difficult for babies to digest, and some brands are high in salt. The best advice is to introduce soy products gradually, in small amounts, after the first two months of weaning. Do not feed your baby nuts or seeds or their products if there is any family history of allergies.

milk and dairy products

Your baby's main source of calcium during her first year is breast milk, infant formula, or follow-on milk. Between six and 12 months she should have at least 500–600ml (18–21fl oz) a day. Cows' milk and other milks, including soy dairy alternatives, can be introduced in small quantities as part of a dish after seven months, when they become a source of protein, calcium, phosphorus, iodine, and vitamin D.

Calcium is essential for healthy bones and teeth and the normal function of all cells, and is vital during this stage, when your baby is growing so fast. Key calcium foods for babies over seven months old include full-fat dairy produce and soy alternatives that are calcium-enriched; finely ground nuts and seeds; dried fruits (in small doses); dark green vegetables, and lentils.

Milk and dairy products, including eggs, can be a good source of iodine, which is required for healthy thyroid function, which affects many other body functions. Other good sources of iodine include butter beans. Vitamin D is essential for the absorption of calcium and the growth and development of strong teeth and bones, and to maintain a healthy immune system. Breastfed babies rely on their stores at birth and later on exposure to sunlight. Vitamin D is naturally found in a few foods – for example, eggs and full-fat milk.

Milk and dairy products are an important source of vitamin B_{12}. A deficiency of B_{12} can lead to anaemia. For their first six months babies get their vitamin B_{12} requirements from breast milk or formula. Once weaning begins they will get their B_{12} from small amounts of dairy products and eggs, and also from fortified foods such as soy formula low-salt yeast extract.

breads, cereals and potatoes

These foods are your baby's main source of carbohydrate. There are two types of carbohydrates: simple (sugars) and complex (starches and fibres). They are the body's primary source of energy. During weaning your baby needs a good supply of energy to sustain her rapid growth and development. After about a month, carbohydrates should form the basis of most meals.

Starches and fibres can be refined or natural. Refined starch foods include baby rice, white bread, and processed breakfast cereals. Baby rice is an ideal first food and can be mixed with breast milk or formula. Cornmeal, sago, or millet can also be given as a thin porridge made with boiled and cooled water, breast milk, or formula. Wheat-based foods, which contain gluten, should not be given before seven months. Highly processed foods, such as biscuits, should not be given to weaning babies as they are often high in saturated fat, sugar, artificial additives, and gluten.

Natural starch foods include potatoes, breakfast cereals, bread, root vegetables, and bananas – potatoes, root vegetables, and bananas can be eaten from six months, whereas cereals and bread cannot be given until seven months. Starch is easily absorbed, so even though it can be bulky, it is easy to ensure your baby will consume enough. However, some starchy foods are also high in fibre, which she cannot tolerate. Too much fibre will fill her up before all her nutritional needs have been met and can hinder her ability to absorb vitamins and minerals. You should never give her bran. The best carbohydrates to introduce early on in weaning are potatoes – ordinary and sweet – and they are easily mixed with protein- or fat-rich foods later on. Bread can be added to purées, or sugar-free muesli, or can be ground and mixed with water, breast milk or formula, or yogurt from eight months. These foods are also important sources of protein and some vitamins, including B_1, B_2, B_3, and B_6 and minerals, particularly zinc. Zinc is important for a healthy immune system. Vegetarian babies can be at risk from zinc deficiency as wholemeal high-fibre foods can inhibit the absorption of zinc, and they tend to eat more of these foods. The best sources of zinc for babies over seven months are full-fat cheese, finely ground sesame and pumpkin seeds, and lentils.

selected foods containing fat and sugar

Fats are an essential part of a healthy diet. They are important during your baby's first year as they provide a concentrated source of energy, needed for her rapid growth and development. Fats allow the body to utilize fat-soluble vitamins A, D, E, and K, and provide essential fatty acids that are vital for a healthy development. All fats are a combination of three types of fatty acids. Saturated fats, such as butter, are solid at room temperature and are sometimes referred to as the 'bad' fats. Hard cheese, cream, and coconut and palm oil are all high in saturated fat. Small amounts of dairy products will provide enough of this kind of fat in your baby's diet.

Monounsaturated and polyunsaturated fats tend to be liquid at room temperature. Unsaturated fats, particularly polyunsaturated fats, are high in omega-3 and omega-6 essential fatty acids. Omega-3 and omega-6 fatty acids are vital for good health, particularly healthy brain development, and the immune and nervous systems. They are predominantly found in oily fish. For vegetarians, the best sources are cold-pressed oils: vegetable oils including olive oil, corn oil, sunflower oil, rapeseed (canola) oil; nuts and their oils (particularly walnuts); seeds (particularly pumpkin seeds and sesame seeds) and their oils; avocados; flax or linseed and their oils. Do not feed nuts or seeds to babies if there is any family history of allergies.

Babies between six and 12 months need around 700–1,000 kilocalories/day. As their stomachs are small they need concentrated sources of energy, so foods containing unsaturated fats are ideal. Try giving your baby high-energy foods such as avocado or pasteurized cheese (from seven months), or add vegetable oil to another food to increase its energy value (for example, add a little olive oil to a vegetable purée). Sugar is not a good source of energy for babies because it provides only empty calories with no nutritional benefits. And it is important not to encourage too sweet a tooth at this stage, as this can be carried into later life. Too much sugar also causes tooth decay. Honey should not be given to babies under 12 months.

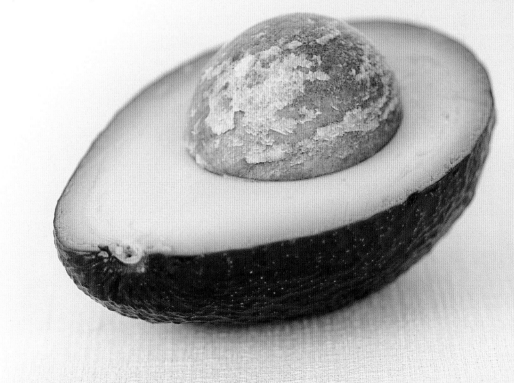

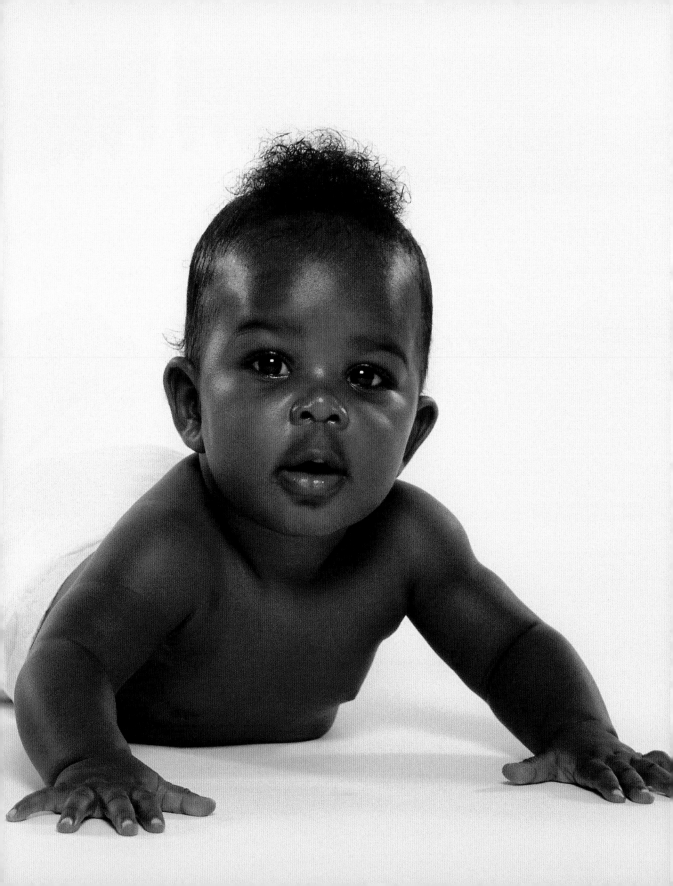

Good nutrition is vital to help your baby's body to function, grow, and repair itself, and to help ensure good health throughout his life. The food you feed your baby during his first year of life will have an impact on his future diet and consequently his future health. Help to teach your baby about good food and give him the best start by breastfeeding for the first six months. Breast milk provides all the food and drink, and so all the nutrients that your baby needs for healthy growth and development until he is six months old. When he is ready to be weaned on to solid foods, offer him fresh, unprocessed 'real' food, cooked simply. Help to teach him about good food right from the word go. If he gets used to the flavour and texture of fresh food from a young age he is more likely to be eating pretty much the same healthy, well-balanced vegetarian diet as the rest of the family by the time he is 12 months old.

your baby's
first year

up to
6 months

World Health Organisation advice

The World Health Organisation (WHO) recommends exclusive breastfeeding for the first six months of your baby's life. Breast milk provides all the food and drink, and so all the nutrients that your baby needs for healthy growth and development until he is six months old. It also contains antibodies that will protect your baby from infection. By breastfeeding your baby, you will be giving him the best possible start in life.

From six months you will need to introduce solid foods – this is known as weaning (see page 41). Breastfed babies can be easier to wean because they have tasted traces of your food in your breast milk. It is still advisable to continue to breastfeed alongside weaning, especially during the first year, because many of the health benefits gained by you and your baby are increased the longer breastfeeding continues. There is evidence to suggest that breastfed babies may be less likely to become obese in later life.

Babies who are exclusively breastfed are less likely to experience gastrointestinal and respiratory infections because breast milk will continue to boost your baby's immune system for as long as it is offered. Breastfeeding can optimize brain development and minimize the chances of neurological problems. There is also evidence that breastfed babies can have higher IQs than bottle-fed babies because of the essential fatty acids and other key nutrients in breast milk, regardless of the genetic make-up of their parents. There are also benefits for you if you breastfeed: you should find it easier to lose the weight you gained during your pregnancy because breastfeeding uses up calories and helps you to burn off excess fat. The longer you breastfeed, the lower the risk you have of developing pre-menopausal breast cancer and ovarian cancer, and breastfeeding may help you to have stronger bones later in life. Also, breastfeeding is practical, it is free, breast milk does not take time to prepare, and it is always at the right temperature – even in the middle of the night.

The WHO carried out extensive research about the optimum duration of exclusive breastfeeding before recommending exclusive breast milk for the first six months. It reviewed 20 independent studies (nine from developing countries and 11 from developed countries). Its findings concluded that breast milk is the best form of nutrition for babies for their first six months of life. Similarly, the Scientific Advisory Committee on Nutrition (SACN) concluded that there are unlikely to be any risks associated with delaying weaning to six months in infants who are either breastfed, mixed fed on breast and infant milk, or fed solely on infant formula milk.

The WHO also recognized that even though six months is the recommended age to introduce solid foods for all normal, healthy babies, whether breastfed, given infant formula, or mixed fed, all babies are individuals and should be treated as such. If you have any concerns about your baby's developmental or nutritional needs, seek advice from your health visitor or family doctor about introducing solid foods. If you are advised to introduce solid foods before six months you will need to be aware of the foods that should be avoided.

It is believed that if solid food is introduced too early this can increase the risk of infections and the development of allergies. There is also some concern that the early introduction of solids can reduce the absorption of nutrients from breast milk. Similarly, the myth has been dispelled that babies need to explore tastes and textures before six months to help with speech development and the acceptance of a wider variety of foods. "Babies can be offered food at an earlier age than six months; however, their oral anatomy, reflex responses, and resulting oral motor function suggest that this is developmentally premature." UK Department of Health

By weaning your baby on to solid foods at around six months you also have the advantage of being able to feed your baby a varied diet more quickly than if you were to wean him at an earlier age. You can increase the amount of solid foods over the next few months so that they become the main part of the baby's diet, with breast or formula milk making up the balance. Your aim should be that, by the time your baby is a year old, he will be eating a varied vegetarian diet (see page 41).

6–9 months

what's happening to my baby?

Your baby will now be more alert, especially visually, and he will take far more notice of things around him. He will begin to be selective about the people around him and may be wary of strangers. He will sleep less during the day and will gradually become more active. He will be more mobile and able to roll over on to his tummy, lift his head, sit unsupported, and perhaps stand while being held or hold on to pieces of furniture. He will be able to wave hello and goodbye, and may even be able to crawl. You will become increasingly aware of his babbling because he starts to make more recognizable sounds, such as 'ga-ga', 'ma-ma', and 'da-da'. Now is a good time to introduce a few simple games: for example, show him a picture of a cow, say 'moo', and watch his response.

eating and drinking

You can now start to introduce your baby to solid foods; this process is known as 'weaning' (see page 41). Your baby's coordination will be much improved, and he will be able to move objects from hand to hand and hand to mouth. His teeth may be developing, and he will quickly learn how to suck from a spoon, eat finger foods, and swallow food successfully. He may show a preference for feeding himself, which means that you can start to introduce soft finger foods. His appetite will increase as he becomes more active, and he will see other people eating and drinking, and want to imitate them. Try to feed him some meals at the same time as the rest of the family eats, so that he feels he belongs and can copy what other family members are doing.

first foods

Because your baby is being weaned at six months he will quite quickly become receptive to a wide range of tastes and textures. However, it is still advisable to feed him a few single purées to start with, to allow him to have a gradual transition from exclusive breast milk to breast milk mixed with solid food. You can then move quickly on to other food because his tastes buds will really develop over the next six to eight weeks. It is important to give your baby lots of different foods at this stage, especially foods with stronger flavours – for example, vegetables such as broccoli, spinach, turnip, and even mildly spiced foods may be accepted, even if only after the third try. After this development period, especially as he becomes more aware, he will have acquired strong preferences for certain foods, and introducing new flavours will become more difficult – particularly if you have fed your baby only ready-prepared baby foods, which are often bland. Different babies develop at different rates, and only you will know at what point your baby is likely to be confident with chewing. At seven to eight months, your baby is likely to progress from puréed to mashed food and finger foods very quickly. In fact he may show a preference for feeding himself quite early into the weaning process. If you do find that he is ready to feed himself, and that he would prefer to do this, you could start to offer him soft finger foods that he will find easy to eat, such as pieces of avocado and banana. Never leave your baby alone while he is eating.

Good first foods include fresh fruit and vegetable purées. Choose fruits and vegetables that will help to boost his immature immune system which fights off infections and diseases. Breast milk is still the primary source of nutrition for your baby, but the nutrients he gets from solids are becoming more important. Give foods that are nutrient-dense and high in energy. If you are considering feeding your baby a vegan diet you should consult your health visitor or family doctor first. The most important nutrients for vegetarian babies during these months include those listed on page 54.

vitamin B$_2$ Good sources include ground wholegrain cereals and green leafy vegetables.

vitamin C A powerful, immune-boosting vitamin that is great for helping to fight colds. It is also essential for assisting iron absorption. Carrots, mangoes, and broccoli are all good early weaning foods and excellent sources of vitamin C.

vitamin D This is made in your baby's skin when he's exposed to sunlight, so make sure that your baby has at least half an hour outside every day, weather permitting. Vegetarian babies can have a little dairy produce, which will boost their vitamin D. Vegan babies should be given vegan margarine, which is fortified with vitamin D.

vitamin E An antioxidant vitamin vital to help protect your baby from diseases that occur later in life. Sweet potatoes and avocados are good sources and great early weaning foods.

betacarotene The body converts betacarotene into vitamin A, which is a good antioxidant.

zinc Essential for a healthy immune system. Good sources for babies of this age include rice and green vegetables, such as peas and spinach.

carbohydrates Foods that are high in carbohydrates, such as bread and pasta, can be added to his diet from six months, but not before three weeks of weaning.

protein A good source of protein will be needed, such as beans, cereals, pulses, finely ground nuts and seeds (do not feed nuts or seeds to babies if there is any history of food allergies), and tofu (from seven months).

iron Especially important, because babies are born with a natural store of this nutrient which becomes depleted at around six months. Good sources include pulses (from seven months) and green vegetables.

calcium Dairy produce can be given in small quantities at this age. Good sources for a vegan diet are green vegetables, chopped dried fruits, ground nuts, and fortified foods such as bread (from seven months).

iodine Good sources include grains and vegetables (from seven months). You may also like to include an iodine supplement. Speak to your family doctor or nutritionist for more information.

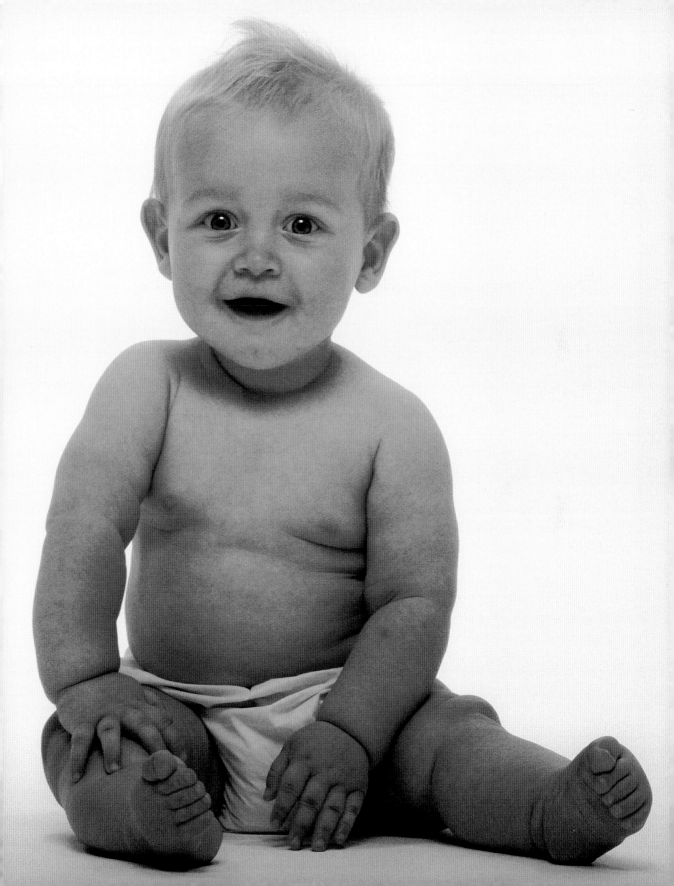

foods to introduce at 7–9 months

It's important to remember that babies develop at different paces, and will learn to chew at different rates, so only you will know when they are ready for new and different foods. They should never be left alone with food at any time. After your baby has been eating single vegetable purées for at least four weeks you can consider introducing the following:

- Puréed cooked pulses, such as lentils, chickpeas, haricot beans, flageolet beans, and kidney beans.
- Wheat or wheat-based foods, such as pasta and sugar-free unrefined cereals.
- Small amounts of full-fat dairy produce, such as natural yogurt, puréed pasteurized cheese, or calcium-enriched soy dairy alternatives to milk, and yogurt.
- Seedless citrus fruits – but mix with other fruits to counteract their sugar and acid content
- Puréed dried fruits can be introduced gradually at nine months – mix with other fruits because they might cause an upset stomach.
- Water, boiled and cooled, as a drink between meals.
- Finely ground nuts and smooth nut butters, assuming there is no family history of nut allergies (see p. 35).
- Small amounts of puréed well-cooked eggs – the yolk must be cooked and not runny.
- Small amounts of cows' milk can be used in dishes – for example, to make a white sauce or custard.

Breast milk or formula milk continues to be the primary source of nutrition for your baby when he is six to nine months old. However, the nutrients that are provided by solid food become more and more important to him, and at seven to nine months you need to establish a routine in which your baby eats three meals a day which include cooled boiled tap water and, later on in this period, finger foods at mealtimes as well as in-between meals.

After a few weeks of weaning you can gradually start to offer breast milk or formula milk as an after-solids drink only. Begin by doing this at breakfast time, when your baby will be at his hungriest and so (hopefully) will eat more solids.

This is also the time for introducing lots of new foods to your baby's diet and increasing the quantity that you give him. Remember, though, that each baby is different and will need to eat varying amounts of food. To a certain extent you will need to follow your baby's direction and use your own initiative when deciding how much to feed him each day.

foods to avoid at 7–9 months

- Cows' milk should not be given as a drink, although small amounts can be used in meals. Milk can be one of the most residue-contaminated foods, so I would always use organic milk.
- Unpasteurized cheese may contain the bacteria listeria, which can cause food poisoning. Avoid all soft cheese (including blue cheese) for your baby's first year.
- Soft-boiled eggs and runny yolks may contain the food-poisoning bacteria salmonella. Babies are far more sensitive than adults to salmonella. Eggs should always be hardboiled.
- Salt cannot be processed by a baby's immature digestive system; it causes dehydration and should not be added to any foods given to babies. A diet high in salt often leads to high blood pressure. Particular foods to avoid at this stage are yeast extracts, such as Marmite or Vegemite, and stock cubes. Most food labels refer to salt as sodium. The salt content is 2.5 times the listed sodium content. Processed foods that are not made specifically for babies, such as pasta sauces and breakfast cereals, should be avoided because they can be high in salt.
- Refined or unrefined sugar provides calories but few nutrients. It's a major cause of tooth decay and can lead to a sweet tooth or health problems such as obesity. It is not necessary to add sugar to your baby's food. Check labels because sugar may be present as sucrose, glucose, fructose, lactose, hydrolyzed starch, invert sugar, and products such as treacle, honey, golden syrup, and corn syrup.
- Never give your baby artificial sweeteners.
- Honey may contain botulism spores, which can cause food poisoning, and this is far more serious in babies than it is in adults. It is also a sugar and can cause the same problems as refined or unrefined sugar. It should not be given to a baby under the age of 12 months
- Avoid excessively hot or spicy foods, which can burn or inflame babies' stomachs.
- Tea and coffee contain tannins that inhibit iron absorption. Babies cannot tolerate caffeine.
- Whole nuts should not be given to children under the age of five because they can cause choking. If there is any history of allergy in your family, avoid nuts, nut products, or foods containing nuts until your child is at least three years old, and seek professional advice from your doctor or state-registered nutritionist.
- Avoid excessively hot spices, such as red chilli powder and cloves, before the age of 12 months. Milder spices, such as coriander, cumin, and cinnamon, can be used sparingly.

10–12 months

what's happening to my baby?

This is the stage at which your baby really begins to appreciate the routine of mealtimes, making him feel more secure and part of the family – especially if you eat as many meals together as possible. His coordination and appreciation of colour and texture will also be developing. Now is the time to give him foods that will help to stimulate his senses and not just his appetite. He will be able to point at objects, pick things up with his finger and thumb, and maybe even put things into and pick them out of his bowl.

At mealtimes your baby will probably be choosing to feed himself, if he hasn't already been doing so. He will particularly enjoy feeding himself finger foods. He will also learn to let go of things deliberately; things may start to get messy, but this is when your baby really begins to learn about and appreciate good food. Get into the habit of giving him foods that you enjoy – my daughter Jasmin's love of spicy food began at about 10 months, when I gave her a little of my favourite Thai green curry.

Your child will now have a sense of humour – even saying 'boo' will make him laugh. He will enjoy playing, especially at bathtime, and hearing you sing nursery rhymes will be a great source of entertainment to him. He may be able to say 'mama' and 'dada', and can indicate what he wants by gesturing instead of crying, both of which will make play more exciting.

Your baby is likely to begin to explore the world on foot by around 11 months, and it is important not to rush this. Often he will move by holding on to pieces of furniture and negotiating small distances between them with a little help from you. He may even be able to stand alone for a few seconds and will gradually learn to walk unaided.

However, it is also at this stage that babies begin to assert their independence by saying 'no'. Your baby will also begin to understand the word 'no' when you say it, but won't necessarily obey it. Try not to get too frustrated. At mealtimes, having smaller amounts of food on the plate often helps; otherwise, just take the food away and don't be tempted to offer sweet alternatives. Try creating interest at mealtimes by involving your baby in the preparation – even if it is only watching you chop carrots. Give food that can easily be held by small fingers – sticks of vegetables, rice cakes, breadsticks, and fingers of cheese, for example, are all great.

At this stage it is important to encourage your baby to eat new things to ensure he is getting a wide range of nutrients. Solid food is just as important as breast milk now as a source of nutrition for your baby.

Adequate energy will be crucial for him as he starts to crawl and move about. Fat will be an essential energy-dense nutrient in his diet. Remember, it's the quality of the fat that matters – try using more unsaturated fats, such as olive oil and avocado.

Foods such as cereals and fresh fruits that are rich in slow-releasing carbohydrates are best for breakfast because they give your baby a steady flow of energy until his next feed. Many mums see all types of sugar as an easy way to give their baby energy; sugar is a carbohydrate, but it gives only short bursts of energy and has little nutritional value, so ideally it should be avoided. Sugar is also a major cause of tooth decay, to which first teeth are susceptible. Too much sugar can lead to health problems, such as obesity, later in life. It is not necessary to add sugar to your baby's food, even when foods are tart: just use other ripe fruits or apple juice to sweeten them.

Protein is essential for the healthy growth of every single one of the body's cells, and it is constantly being used and replaced. Because your baby is growing so rapidly, he will need more protein in relation to his weight than an adult. Good vegetarian sources of protein for babies at this stage include full-fat dairy products, well-cooked eggs, beans, pulses, soy products such as tofu, and calcium-enriched soy drinks and yogurt alternatives. While protein from animal sources is generally a complete protein, vegetarian and vegan diets need a combination of cereals, pulses, and vegetables to get complete protein because no non-animal source, except tofu, is a complete protein (see page 22).

To help keep your baby's bowel movements regular, begin to introduce a little fibre into his diet. His digestive system is still immature and he will not be able to cope with the bulky fibre found in brown rice, wholewheat, and bran. Instead, include foods such as peas, fruit, and vegetable juices, which are easier for his system to tolerate.

Also ensure he drinks enough liquid because too little fluid is one of the main causes of constipation in babies. Cooled, boiled water from a cup should be given between feeds. Encourage your baby to drink most of his feed at this stage from a cup because this is recommended for the development of your baby's healthy teeth and at this stage he should be able to hold a cup himself.

The main aim of this stage of weaning is, by the age of 12 months, to be able to include him at all family meals and not have to cook separate meals for him, although obviously you will have to chop or mash his food as necessary. Don't add salt during cooking and introduce new foods in small quantities with something familiar so that your baby does not feel overwhelmed.

foods to introduce at 10–12 months

It's important to remember that babies develop at different paces, and they should never be left alone with food at any time.

- As the amount of solid food in your baby's diet increases, he will need some fibre to help keep his bowel movements regular. Soluble fibre, found in foods such as peas, fruit, and vegetable juices, is sufficient because his immature digestive system will not be able to cope with the bulky fibre found in brown rice and wholewheat.
- At least one baby portion of protein should be given each day – see page 16 for examples of vegetarian protein-rich foods

A 10-month-old baby will begin to appreciate the routine of mealtimes, making him feel more secure and part of the family – especially if you eat as many meals together as possible. Three key changes to a baby's diet take place at 10 months. The first is his milk intake: it is important to reduce this in order to allow more room in his small tummy for solid food. Often parents are tempted to give milk when a baby of this age cries. Try to give solids instead – they will keep him satisfied for longer as he becomes more active. But be sure to give your baby plenty of liquids besides milk, such as water and juice, to avoid constipation.

The second key change is the balance of nutrition. Immune-boosting foods continue to be important, but the real focus is on strength. Your baby needs more starch, protein, sugar, and fats to enable him to build up the strength to crawl and walk.

The third key change is volume. Your baby is likely to start really enjoying food now. His coordination and appreciation of colour and texture will be developing, so try to encourage him to eat well by giving him lots of variety. However, it is also at this stage that babies begin to assert their independence by saying 'no'. Again, try not to get too frustrated over this: having smaller amounts of food on the plate often helps prevent it, otherwise, just take the food away and don't be tempted to offer your baby sweet alternatives.

foods to avoid at 10–12 months

- Cows' milk or soy milk as a drink.
- If there is any history of allergy in your family, avoid nuts, nut products, or foods containing nuts until your child is at least three years old, and seek professional advice from your doctor or state-registered nutritionist. Whole nuts should never be given to children under the age of five because there is a risk of choking.
- Unpasteurized cheese may contain the bacteria listeria, which can cause food poisoning. Babies are more sensitive to this bacteria than adults.
- Too much salt can't be processed by a baby's immature digestive system: it causes dehydration. A diet high in salt often leads to high blood pressure later. Particular foods to avoid at this stage are yeast extracts, such as Marmite or Vegemite, and stock cubes.
- Refined or unrefined sugar provides calories, but has little nutritional value. Always give sweet things, such as fruit, at mealtimes so the acid that damages teeth is diluted – cheese is particularly good at doing this. Check food labels carefully because sugar may be present as sucrose, glucose, fructose, lactose, hydrolysed starch, invert sugar, and products such as treacle, honey, and syrup.
- Never use artificial sweeteners.
- Avoid honey until your baby is 12 months old: it may contain botulism spores that can cause food poisoning.
- Excessively hot or spicy foods can burn or inflame babies' stomachs.
- Tea and coffee contain tannins and inhibit iron absorption. Caffeine is a stimulant, which babies cannot tolerate. Most fizzy drinks also contain caffeine and should be avoided.
- Soft-boiled eggs and runny yolks may contain the food-poisoning bacteria salmonella. Babies are far more sensitive than adults to salmonella. Eggs should always be hardboiled.

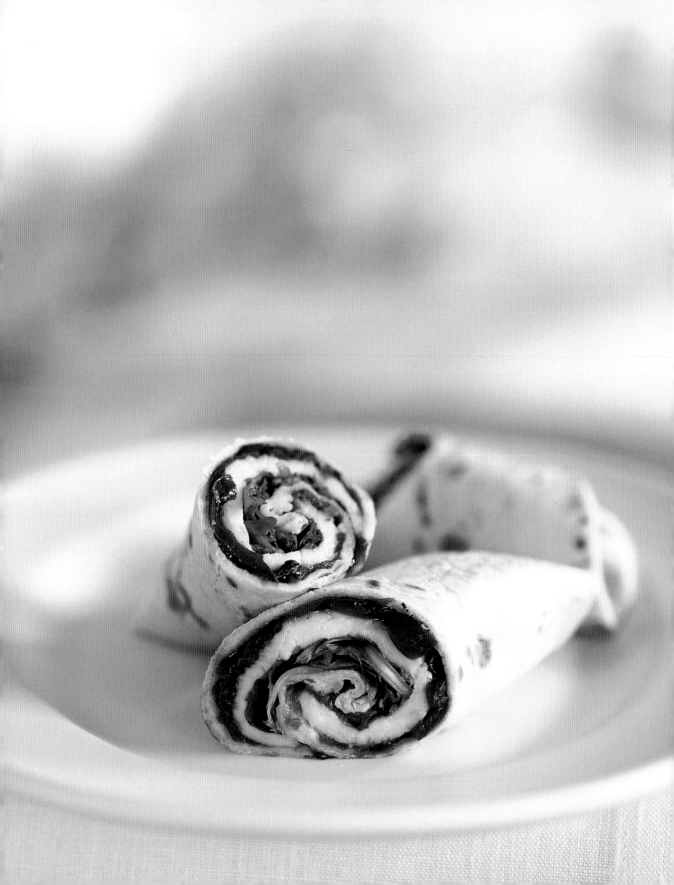

During your pregnancy, your baby is completely dependent on you for the nutrients that she needs to grow and develop. It is therefore important that you eat a well-balanced vegetarian diet. To help you, this chapter contains lots of easy recipes for breakfasts, lunches, and suppers. It can be tough when you are pregnant and feeling tired, so on the whole, the recipes are quick. The few recipes that take a little longer can be prepared in advance and kept in the refrigerator or popped in the freezer.

Be prepared to experiment a little with your food to make sure that you eat as many different foods as possible. For example, add handfuls of toasted seeds to soups or salads. Keep an eye on the nutrients that you need (see pages 16–29) and enjoy the recipes during both pregnancy and breastfeeding. Just one last thing, try to eat supper a couple of hours before bedtime to give your body time to digest the food before you go to sleep. This should help you to have a better night's sleep and may alleviate any indigestion problems.

pregnancy
recipes

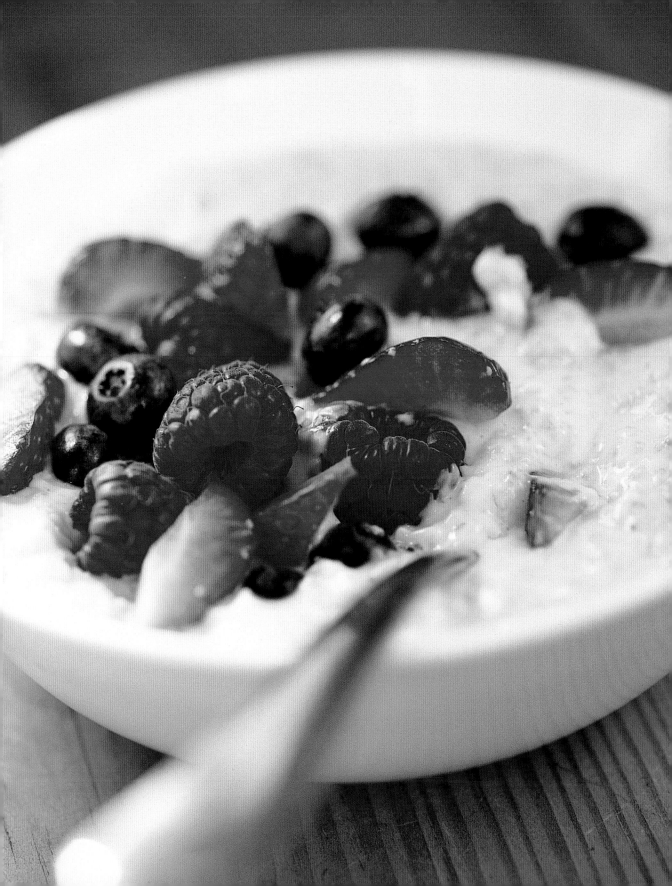

vegetarian pregnancy
breakfasts

creamy coconut porridge

makes: 2 portions

storage: best eaten immediately

handful of blueberries, picked over
handful of strawberries, hulled
1 tbsp lime juice
200ml (7fl oz) coconut milk
200ml (7fl oz) water
200g (7oz) porridge oats

This is delicious on a cold winter morning: the porridge is rich and creamy, a contrast to the fresh fruits. Oats are a great source of carbohydrate and fibre, and provide an energy-packed breakfast that should keep you satisfied for a while – at least until the middle of the morning! Coconut milk makes a welcome change from cow's milk and gives the porridge a wonderful subtle nutty flavour and rich creamy texture. (Do not eat nut products if there is any family history of allergies.)

1   Put the strawberries and blueberries into a bowl, then sprinkle them with the lime juice.
2   Put the coconut milk and water into a saucepan and bring to the boil. Reduce to a gentle simmer and add the oats. Stir constantly over a low heat until the mixture thickens – about 5 minutes.
3   Pour into a bowl and top with the fruit.

strawberry shake

makes: 2 portions

storage: best drunk immediately, or up to 1–2 days in the refrigerator

200g (7oz) strawberries, hulled
1 large ripe banana, peeled and
    chopped
fortified soy drink (milk
    alternative), enough to make a
    good consistency
a little unrefined sugar, to taste
    (optional)

Strawberries are a good source of betacarotene, which helps to boost the immune system. Bananas are a good source of folic acid and fortified soy drink provides protein.

1   Throw the fruit into a food processor or blender with a little soy drink and whizz until smooth.
2   Add enough milk to make a smooth, thick (but not too thick) shake. Add sugar to taste, if liked.

mango and melon smoothie

makes: 2 portions

storage: best drunk immediately, or whizz fruits and add water just before drinking

1 mango
½ melon, such as ogen or cantaloupe, peeled and deseeded
sparkling water (optional)

A whole mango provides more than the daily requirement of vitamin C. Melons provide folic acid, which helps to prevent birth defects.

1 Cut the mango either side of the stone, peel off the flesh, and put it into a food processor or blender.

2 Add the melon flesh and whiz until smooth. Add sparkling water if you want to dilute it slightly.

dried fruit compote

makes: 4 portions

storage: up to 2–3 days in the refrigerator

200ml (7fl oz) apple juice
200ml (7fl oz) orange juice
350g (12oz) mixed dried fruit, such as pears, peaches, prunes, apricots, and figs
handful of raisins
½ tsp ground cinnamon
1 cinnamon stick

Cooking the dried fruit in juice makes it really plump and sweet. Choose fruit that you like – I used pears, peaches, figs, etc. Alternatively, you could use a bag of mixed dried fruit. This compote will keep for a few days, covered and stored in the refrigerator. Mixed dried fruit is a good source of iron and folic acid. Apple and orange juice are both good sources of vitamin C, which improves iron absorption in the body.

1 Put all the ingredients into a pan and bring to the boil.

2 Remove the cinnamon stick.

3 Remove from the heat and leave to cool.

mixed fruit with toasted oats

makes: 2 portions

storage: best eaten immediately, or up to 1–2 days in the refrigerator

40g (1½oz) organic oats
1 large ripe mango, peeled, pitted, and chopped
6 strawberries, hulled and sliced
juice of ½ lime
100g (3¾oz) natural Greek yogurt
runny honey, to taste

This is an easy way to incorporate more fresh fruit into your diet. Toasting the oats gives them a wonderful crunch, and they will help to keep your energy levels up during the morning.

1 Lightly toast the oats in a dry frying pan until lightly golden. Set aside.
2 Toss the fruit with the lime juice and put into two dishes.
3 Top with yogurt and the toasted oats. Drizzle with honey.

fresh fruit salad

makes: 2 portions

storage: best eaten immediately, or keep fruit and sauce separately for up to 2–3 days in the refrigerator

a selection of fresh fruit of your choice, such as 1 mango, 1 nectarine, and 1 papaya, prepared and cut into chunks
natural full-fat yogurt
sunflower seeds, to serve

for the raspberry sauce:
150g (5½oz) raspberries or mixed berries, frozen or fresh
1–2 tsp golden caster sugar
squeeze of lime or lemon juice

Fresh fruit is a good source of fibre and vitamin C, which helps the body with digestion and absorption of iron. Yogurt provides calcium, which helps with the formation of bones. Another delicious winning combination is a mixture of melon, papaya, and fresh basil or mint, with a little maple syrup drizzled over the top.

1 Make the sauce: put all the ingredients in a heavy-based saucepan and simmer until the raspberries have turned to a pulp. Taste for sweetness, adding a little extra caster sugar if neccessary. Leave to cool.
2 Scatter your chosen fresh fruit over two plates and drizzle the cooled raspberry sauce over the top, finishing with a dollop of yogurt and a sprinkling of sunflower seeds.

nutty fruit bar

makes: 15 bars

storage: in an airtight container for up to 2 weeks

50g (1¾oz) butter
25g (1oz) golden caster sugar
75g (2½oz) golden syrup
250g (9oz) jumbo rolled oats
25g (1oz) pumpkin seeds, toasted
50g (1¾oz) Brazil nuts, chopped
  and toasted
40g (1½oz) dried apricots, roughly
  chopped
40g (1½oz) dried mango, cut into
  small pieces
1 tbsp sesame seeds, toasted

Once you have made these, you can just grab one as and when you choose. They will keep in an airtight container or in the freezer. These bars are packed with goodness: the oats provide folic acid, and the seeds and nuts are good sources of zinc, calcium, and iron. (Do not eat nuts if there is any family history of allergies.)

1 Grease a 20cm (9 inch) square tin. Preheat the oven to 180°C/350°F/gas mark 4. Put the butter, sugar, and syrup into a pan and heat gently until the butter is melted.

2 Add the remaining ingredients and mix well. Tip into the greased tin and bake in the oven for 25-30 minutes.

3 Mark into squares and leave to cool in the tin. Cut and store in an airtight container.

bircher-style muesli

makes: 2 portions

storage: best eaten immediately

2 tbsp porridge oats
6 tbsp milk
natural full-fat yogurt, to taste
runny honey, to taste
juice of ½ lemon
2 fresh peaches
2 small apples, such as Cox's
  orange pippin
150g (5½oz) toasted chopped nuts,
  such as hazelnuts, almonds, or
  walnuts

Bircher muesli is based on whole oats, grains, nuts, milk, and fruit. It was invented by Dr Bircher-Benner, a Swiss physician and pioneer of food reform. Unlike most shop-bought muesli, the oats in this recipe are soaked in milk or water before being mixed with the other ingredients. The result is the oats are slightly creamy, with a soft, almost cooked texture. You can change the type of fruit depending on what's in season. (Do not eat nuts if there is any family history of allergies.)

1 Put the oats and milk into a bowl and leave to soak in the refrigerator overnight – if you prefer a slight crunch, mix them just 10–15 minutes before you are going to eat them.

2 Stir in the yogurt and honey, to taste, and the lemon juice.

3 Stone the peaches and cut into slices. Grate the apple. Quickly but gently mix the fruit into the muesli. Add the nuts and serve immediately.

poached egg on a toasted roll

makes: 2 portions

storage: best eaten immediately

2 large free-range eggs
2 seeded bread rolls
small knob of butter

Do make sure that you choose either free-range or organic eggs – not only will they taste better, but they will also be better for you and are less likely to have salmonella. Once you have mastered cooking a good poached egg, you can serve them on top of salads for a simple protein-packed lunch.

1   Fill a shallow frying pan with water and bring up to simmering point.
2   Crack an egg into a cup and pour into the water. Repeat with the second egg. Simmer very gently for 5 minutes, or until the white is set and the yolk is firm, basting the top with water as it cooks.
3   Lift the eggs out with a slotted spoon and drain briefly on kitchen paper.
4   Meanwhile, slice the rolls in half and toast them. Spread with the butter. Divide between two plates and top each with an egg. Serve immediately.

sweetcorn fritters

makes: 4–5 portions (20 fritters)

storage: best eaten immediately

2 tbsp olive oil
1 red onion, peeled and finely
  chopped
150g (5½oz) plain flour
1 tsp baking powder
pinch of salt
¼ tsp paprika
2 large free-range eggs
100ml (3½fl oz) full-fat milk
250g (9oz) sweetcorn, frozen, fresh
  or tinned (if using frozen, thaw
  first)
½ red pepper, deseeded and finely
  chopped
large handful of flat-leaf parsley or
  coriander, chopped

These do take a little while to make – especially when compared to normal breakfast fodder, such as a bowl of cereal – so they may be best kept for a lazy weekend brunch or lunch. The fritters are delicious served with some grilled tomatoes. Alternatively, if you want to add a little more protein to your meal, serve with poached eggs.

1   Heat 1 tbsp of the oil in a frying pan and sauté the onion for approximately 5 minutes or until soft.
2   Sieve the flour, baking powder, salt, and paprika into a large bowl.
3   Lightly whisk the eggs and milk together in a jug.
4   Make a well in the centre of the flour mixture and gradually stir in the egg mixture. Whisk until you have a thick, smooth batter.
5   Add the onion, corn, peppers, and parsley and quickly stir everything together.
6   Heat the remaining oil in a large non-stick frying pan. Drop 1–2 tbsp of batter into the pan for each fritter. Cook for about 3 minutes, then carefully flip over and cook the other side. Transfer to a serving plate and serve with grilled tomatoes.

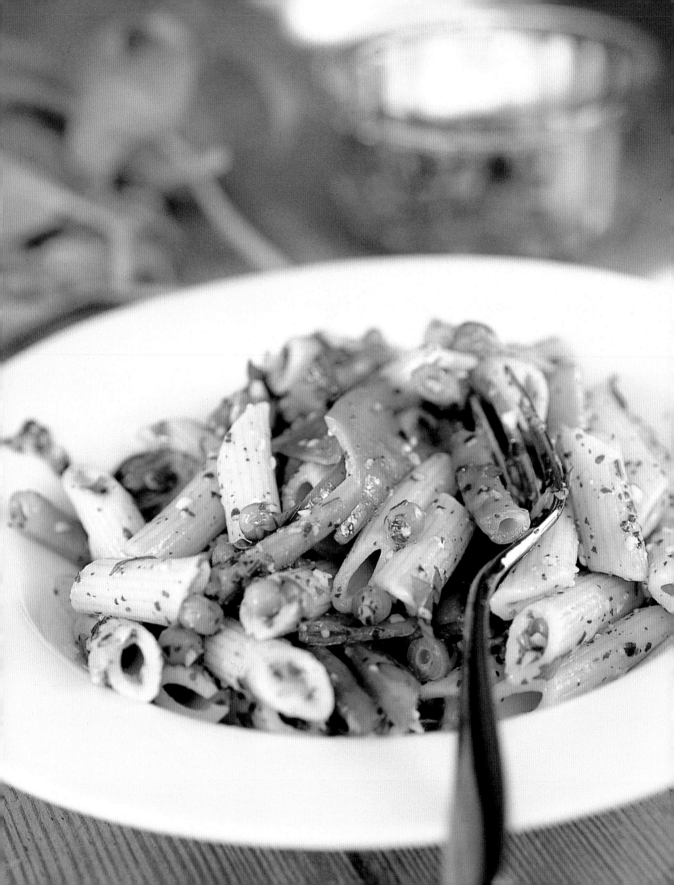

vegetarian pregnancy
lunches

pasta with green beans and pesto

makes: 4 portions

storage: best eaten immediately

500g (1lb) penne or other pasta of
  your choice
200g (7oz) thin green beans
200g (7oz) peas or petits pois
4-5 tbsp pesto sauce
large handful of fresh flat-leaf
  parsley or basil leaves, chopped
  (tear the basil)
grated vegetarian Parmesan-style
  cheese, to serve
salad, to serve

This sort of lunch is simple and quick to make, and tastes delicious.
Use any fresh green vegetables that you have to hand; if asparagus is in season,
try adding a few spears. The vegetables will provide you with vitamins and
minerals, the pasta with some carbohydrate and the nuts in the pesto are a
great source of protein. (Do not eat nuts if there is any family history of
allergies.)

1 Bring a large pan of water to the boil and cook the pasta until *al dente*. Drain.
2 Meanwhile, put the green beans and peas in a steamer and steam over the pasta
    for a few minutes until just cooked – the beans should still have 'bite'.
3 Add the pesto, green vegetables and herbs to the pasta and mix everything
    together. Sprinkle over the grated cheese. Serve immediately with a big bowl of
    salad.

tortilla wraps

makes: 3–4 portions

storage: best eaten immediately or up
to 1–2 days in the refrigerator

2 tbsp olive oil
3 red onions, peeled and finely
  sliced
1 tbsp soft brown sugar
2–3 tsp balsamic vinegar
50g (1¾oz) wild rocket
5 flour tortillas
200g (7oz) vegetarian mozzarella,
  thinly sliced

Be creative with other fillings; tortillas are great with lots of different
flavours. Try cheeses, pestos, and roasted tomatoes. There is a fine line
between too much filling and not quite enough – if you are too generous,
the wraps don't stay neatly rolled, but skimp and you feel slightly cheated.
Mozzarella is a very good source of calcium, which helps to keep bones
strong. Wild rocket provides iron and folic acid, which aid in your body's
growth and development.

1 Heat the oil in a frying pan, add the onions and cook gently for 15 minutes,
    until starting to caramelize. Add the sugar and balsamic vinegar. Cook for
    another 10 minutes, until the onions are sweet and sticky.
2 Lay the rocket on the tortillas, arrange a few slices of mozzarella strips in the
    middle, then cover with a layer of caramelized onions.
3 Roll up the tortillas and wrap in cling film. Refrigerate for at least 30 minutes
    before serving. Remove the cling film, cut each wrap in half and serve.

'anything goes' salad

makes: 3–4 portions

storage: best eaten immediately, or up to 1–2 days in the refrigerator (but keep dressing separate)

handful of sunflower seeds
125g (4½oz) baby spinach leaves, washed and dried
handful of cherry tomatoes, quartered
handful of radishes, sliced
2 small cooked beetroot, peeled and diced
hard pasteurized vegetarian cheese, to serve
fresh crusty bread, to serve

for the dressing:
handful of mint, finely chopped
2 cloves garlic, peeled and crushed
1 tsp runny honey
½–1 tsp Dijon mustard, to taste
sea salt and ground black pepper
2 tbsp red wine vinegar
4 tbsp extra virgin olive oil

Choose your favourite salad ingredients and add to the bowl – as long as you add some spinach. This is great served with cheese and fresh crusty bread. There are quite a few benefits from the ingredients in this salad, depending on what you choose to throw in. To give you an idea: sunflower seeds contain magnesium, which is involved in producing energy; spinach is great for iron, which is essential to the development and growth of an unborn child; tomatoes are a good source of vitamin C, which assists in the absorption of iron; and beetroot is a good source of folic acid, which helps to reduce risks of spina bifida in the early stages of pregnancy.

1 Put the sunflower seeds into a dry frying pan and heat gently for a few minutes. Transfer to a large bowl.
2 Add the baby spinach leaves, cherry tomatoes, radishes and beetroots to the sunflower seeds.
3 Put the dressing ingredients into a screw-top jar, replace the lid, and shake well to mix. Pour the dressing over the salad and toss everything together. Serve with chunks of hard cheese and slices of fresh crusty bread.

chickpea salad

makes: 4 portions

storage: up to 2–3 days in the refrigerator (but keep dressing separate)

½ cucumber
2 x 400g tins chickpeas, drained and rinsed
75g (2½oz) sunblush tomatoes or cherry tomatoes, finely chopped

for the dressing:
1 tsp cumin seeds, dry-fried and ground
2 tbsp natural full-fat yogurt
handful of mint leaves, finely sliced
sea salt and freshly ground black pepper, to taste

This is quick and easy to make, and tastes fabulous. Cumin has quite a powerful flavour – add more or less to suit your taste. Chickpeas provide protein, and cucumber is a source of folic acid, which is essential in the manufacture of amino acids and red blood cells. Tomatoes are a good source of vitamin C, which strengthens the body's immune system.

1 Cut the cucumber in half lengthways, scoop out the seeds, and cut the flesh into small pieces or strips.
2 Put the chickpeas into a bowl and add the cucumber and tomatoes.
3 Mix together the dressing ingredients and pour over the salad. Toss everything together and serve.

bruschetta

makes: 1 portion

storage: best eaten immediately

for the bruschetta:
1 small part-cooked ciabatta loaf
1 clove garlic, peeled

for the cannellini beans:
75g (2½oz) tinned cannellini beans,
  drained and rinsed
1 clove garlic, peeled and crushed
zest and juice of ½–1 unwaxed lemon
2–3 tbsp extra virgin olive oil
6 basil leaves
sea salt and freshly ground black
  pepper
2 tbsp freshly grated vegetarian
  Parmesan-style cheese

for the artichoke:
handful of cooked artichoke hearts
  in oil, drained
squeeze of lemon juice
freshly ground black pepper
2 tbsp finely grated vegetarian
  Parmesan-style cheese
handful of dark-green salad leaves

Cook the ciabatta loaf according to the pack instructions. Slice thickly and arrange on a baking tray. Drizzle with olive oil and return to the hot oven for a few minutes until crisp and golden. Turn over and cook for a few minutes on the other side. Rub each side with garlic. Munch on these with one of the following toppings. Beans are a great source of fibre and protein. Artichokes supply both phosphorus and iron, and are also good for the digestion.

smashed cannellini beans with lemon

1 Mash the beans, garlic, lemon zest and juice, olive oil, and basil in a bowl, or whizz in a food processor or blender.
2 Season with salt and pepper and spread on to the toasted ciabatta. Top with the cheese to serve.

artichoke, lemon and cheese

1 Lightly mash the artichokes, then add the lemon juice and pepper, and mix.
2 Spoon the artichoke on to the ciabatta, and top with the cheese. Eat with fresh green salad leaves.

pea soup

makes: 6 portions

storage: soup lasts up to 2–3 days in the refrigerator, or up to 3 months in the freezer

1 tbsp olive oil, plus extra for
  drizzling
1 large onion, peeled and finely
  chopped
1 clove garlic, peeled and sliced
750g (1lb 11oz) frozen peas
1 litre (1¾ pints) vegetable stock
handful of mint leaves
75g (2½oz) vegetarian Parmesan-
  style cheese, grated

Served with Parmesan-style cheese, mint, and olive oil, this is the perfect soup for when you have no fresh vegetables in the house. Freeze any leftover soup in plastic bags and heat through as and when needed. Peas provide protein, helping the body with growth and development. They also contain folic acid, which can help to prevent birth defects.

1 Heat the oil in a large saucepan and sauté the onion and garlic. Add two-thirds of the peas, the stock, and the mint, reserving some leaves for scattering. Cover and bring to the boil, then simmer for 5 minutes.
2 Purée the mixture in a food processor or blender. Return to the pan, add the remaining peas and stock, and simmer for 5 minutes.
3 Pour into warmed soup bowls, spoon the cheese into the middle of each bowl, scatter over the reserved mint, and drizzle with the extra olive oil.
4 Leave to cool completely. Pour into freezer-proof containers and freeze. Thaw completely before heating through in a saucepan.

avocado and pepper tortilla pizzas

makes: 3 pizzas

storage: best eaten immediately

1 red pepper, halved and deseeded
1 large avocado, halved and stone
  removed
2–3 spring onions
1 red chilli, deseeded
3 flour tortillas
6 tbsp tomato purée
handful of cherry tomatoes, sliced
handful of black olives, pitted and
  sliced
75g (2½oz) vegetarian Cheddar
  cheese, grated

other topping ideas:
thinly sliced tomatoes, wilted
  spinach, and grated vegetarian
  Parmesan-style cheese
sliced tomatoes, grated cheese,
  olives, and finely chopped chilli

This is a very quick and easy way to eat a few more vegetables. Flour tortillas make great pizza bases (as long as you like them thin and crispy), and they come in a multitude of flavours – for example, garlic and coriander. Try other toppings to suit your taste. Vegetarian mozzarella and sweetcorn are scrummy. Red peppers and chillies are an excellent source of vitamin C, which is essential for growth and development. Avocados provide vitamin E, which helps to maintain healthy skin, and flour tortillas are a source of carbohydrates.

1 Preheat the grill to high. Thinly slice the red pepper. Cut the avocado in half and remove the stone. Peel and thinly slice the flesh. Thinly slice the spring onions and the chilli diagonally.

2 Spread each tortilla with 1–2 tablespoons tomato purée. scatter over the pepper, avocado, tomatoes, spring onions, chilli, and olives, and top each with some grated cheese.

3 Grill for 3–5 minutes, until the tortillas are crisp and golden and the cheese has completely melted.

fruity nutty bread

makes: 1kg (2lb) loaf

storage: up to 1 week in an airtight container

2 tbsp sunflower oil
350g (12¼oz) plain flour
150g (5½oz) wholemeal flour
1 tsp sea salt
1 tsp cream of tartar
1 tsp baking soda
1 tsp baking powder
100g (3¾oz) mixed nuts, toasted
  and roughly chopped
100g (3¾oz) sunflower seeds, plus
  extra for sprinkling
100g (3¾oz) dried apricots,
  roughly chopped
250ml (9fl oz) natural full-fat
  yogurt
25ml (1fl oz) full-fat milk
runny honey

This is a very quick yeast-free bread. It is delicious cut into slices and served with a really fruity jam, or mashed banana and cinnamon. (Do not eat nuts if there is any family history of allergies.)

1 Preheat the oven to 180°C/350°F/gas mark 4. Grease a 1kg (2lb) loaf tin with half the oil. Sieve the flours, salt, cream of tartar, baking soda, and baking powder together in a large bowl. Stir in the nuts, sunflower seeds, and apricots.

2 Mix together the yogurt, milk, honey, and the remaining 1 tbsp oil. Stir into the dry ingredients and mix to form a soft dough. Spoon the dough into the oiled tin. Sprinkle the extra sunflower seeds over the top.

3 Bake in the oven for 1 hour – you may need to cover the loaf with greaseproof paper after 40 minutes to prevent it from browning too much.

Italian bean and vegetable soup

makes: 4 portions

storage: keep the pesto in an airtight jar for up to a week in the refrigerator; soup lasts up to 2–3 days in the refrigerator

2 tbsp olive oil
2 onions, peeled and chopped
2 cloves garlic, peeled and chopped
1 leek, finely sliced
2 sprigs of fresh rosemary
400g tin cannellini beans, drained and rinsed
6 ripe tomatoes, finely chopped
1.2 litres (42fl oz) vegetable stock
125g (4½oz) peas
125g (4½oz) French beans
1 courgette, cut into small dice
2 tbsp flat-leaf parsley, chopped
salt and ground black pepper

for the pesto:
2 cloves garlic, peeled and crushed
40g (1½oz) pine nuts, chopped
100g (3¾oz) fresh basil leaves
50ml (2fl oz) olive oil
50g (1¾oz) vegetarian Parmesan-style cheese

If broad beans are in season, add a few handfuls to your soup, for that matter, you can add any green vegetables you fancy. The pesto will keep for a few days in a jar in the refrigerator, and it is ideal for mixing with pasta or swirling through mash. (Do not eat nuts if there is any family history of allergies.)

1 To make the soup, heat the oil in a large heavy-based saucepan, add the onions and sauté for 5 minutes. Add the garlic, leek, and rosemary, then fry gently for 10 minutes, or until softened but not coloured.

2 Add the cannellini beans, tomatoes, stock, peas and beans (ends trimmed, and halved), bring to the boil, and simmer for 10 minutes.

3 Add the courgette and parsley, and cook for another 5 minutes. Season to taste and remove the rosemary.

4 Make the pesto: pound the garlic with the nuts using a pestle and mortar. Add the basil leaves, a handful at a time, alternating with the oil. When all the leaves are ground to a smooth texture, stir in the remaining oil and the cheese, and season to taste.

5 Serve the soup with spoonfuls of pesto on top.

red pepper hummus

makes: 4 portions

storage: keep the hummus in an airtight container in the refrigerator for up to 5 days

for the hummus:
1 red pepper, halved and deseeded
2 x 400g tins chickpeas, drained and rinsed
2 garlic cloves, peeled and chopped
juice of 1 lemon
4 tbsp olive oil
50ml (2fl oz) warm water
1 tbsp tahini paste

to serve:
1 ripe avocado
4 pitta breads
½ lettuce, sliced

I once read a wonderful sentence in a nutrition book: "If the soya bean is the king of beans then the chickpea is without question the queen." I particularly like chickpeas, partly because they are so versatile: they are great whizzed into soups, added to casseroles or made into dips such as hummus, and they are delicious eaten on their own or added to salads.

1 Preheat the grill to high. Put the pepper halves, cut sides down, on a baking sheet and grill the peppers until blackened and soft all over. Put into a plastic bag, tie the end and leave to cool – the steam will make the peppers easier to peel. Remove the pepper from the bag and peel off the skin.

2 Put all the hummus ingredients into a food processor and whizz until smooth. Season to taste.

3 Peel, pit, and slice the avocado. Spoon some hummus into a pitta and add some fresh avocado and lettuce. Serve immediately.

sweet potatoes with spinach

Once your sweet potatoes are cooking, all you have to do is mix together the spinach and yogurt.

makes: 4 portions

storage: best eaten immediately

4 large sweet potatoes
2 tbsp olive oil
2 cloves garlic, peeled and crushed
425g (15oz) fresh leaf spinach,
  thoroughly washed and chopped
600g (1lb 5oz) natural full-fat
  yogurt
1 tbsp lemon juice
freshly ground black pepper
handful of fresh coriander leaves,
  chopped

1 Preheat the oven to 200°C/400°F/gas mark 6. Cut a few slits in the potatoes and rub them all over with 1 tbsp oil. Bake for 1 hour: the potatoes should be soft when pierced with a knife.
2 Heat the remaining 1 tbsp oil in a wok or large frying pan, add the garlic, and sauté for 1 minute until soft. Add the spinach and wilt for 1 minute. Take off the heat.
3 Add the yogurt to the spinach and season with the lemon juice and freshly ground black pepper.
4 Cut a slit in each potato, top with the yogurt mixture, and scatter over the fresh coriander.

Mediterranean couscous

Haloumi cheese can be quite salty, so taste before you season. (Do not eat nuts if there is any family history of allergies.)

makes: 4 portions

storage: best eaten immediately, or up to 2–3 days in the refrigerator

200g (7oz) couscous
200ml (7fl oz) boiling water or
  vegetable stock
6 tbsp olive oil
juice of 1 lemon
1 clove garlic, peeled and finely
  chopped
½ tsp seeded mustard
2 tbsp finely chopped flat-leaf
  parsley
freshly ground black pepper
10cm (4 inch) piece of cucumber,
  halved, deseeded and cut into
  small dice
2 ripe plum tomatoes, halved,
  deseeded and cut into small dice
4 tbsp toasted pine nuts
50g (1¾oz) black olives, pitted
  and chopped
350g (12oz) vegetarian haloumi
2 tbsp plain flour

1 Put the couscous into a bowl. Pour over the boiling water or stock. Cover and leave to sit in a warm place for at least 20 minutes.
2 Fluff up the couscous with a fork and put into a serving bowl. Mix together 4 tbsp olive oil with the lemon juice, garlic, mustard, and parsley. Season with black pepper. Pour half of the dressing over the couscous. Add the cucumber, tomato, pine nuts, and olives, and mix gently.
3 Meanwhile prepare the haloumi. Cut into 8 slices and lay on absorbent kitchen paper. Heat the remaining oil in a frying pan over a high heat.
4 Put the flour on to a plate and season with freshly ground black pepper. Press each piece of haloumi into the seasoned flour, then fry for 1 minute, until golden. Flip them over with a palette knife, and fry the other side.
5 Serve the couscous with the fried haloumi and with the remaining dressing in a jug.

roasted tomato soup

makes: 4 portions

storage: soup lasts up to 2–3 days in the refrigerator, or up to 3 months in the freezer

1kg (2lb 3oz) ripe tomatoes, preferably plum, halved lengthways
1 red onion, peeled and cut into 8 wedges
1 small carrot, peeled and thickly sliced
2 cloves garlic, peeled and sliced
small sprig of rosemary
4 tbsp olive oil
freshly ground black pepper
1 litre (1¾ pints) vegetable stock
sea salt, to taste
1 tsp soft brown sugar, to taste (optional)
1–2 tsp red wine vinegar, to taste (optional)

for the pumpkin seeds:
100g (3¾oz) pumpkin seeds
2 tsp paprika
drizzle of olive oil

If you find this is too tart add a little more sugar. Alternatively, if it is sweet try adding a little red wine vinegar. Roast more pumpkin seeds and keep in an airtight container for up to two weeks; they make a great quick snack and are perfect for helping to keep your intestines healthy. If you like silken tofu, add some to the soup for a little extra protein.

1 Preheat the oven to 200°C/400°F/gas mark 6. Put the tomatoes, onion, carrot, garlic, and rosemary into a large roasting tin. Pour over the olive oil. Use your hands to mix everything together so all the tomatoes are covered in oil, then season with black pepper.

2 Roast for 1 hour or until the onion is soft and the tomato skins have split.

3 Meanwhile scatter the pumpkin seeds on a baking tray or sheet, and sprinkle over the paprika. Drizzle with oil and season well. Roast in the oven, alongside the tomato mixture, for 10 minutes, turning once.

4 Remove the rosemary and tip all the vegetables into a blender or food processor. Add enough of the stock to allow you to purée the mixture until there are no big lumps.

5 Pour the purée into a saucepan, add the remaining stock, and season to taste with sea salt and freshly ground black pepper. Add the sugar or red wine vinegar, if using. Serve in bowls with a drizzle of oil and a spoonful of toasted pumpkin seeds.

cream cheese and spinach wrap

makes: 2 portions

storage: best eaten immediately, or up to 1–2 days in the refrigerator

2 flour tortillas
4 tbsp full-fat cream cheese
8–10 sunblush tomatoes or cherry tomatoes, chopped
½ red pepper, deseeded and finely chopped
2 handfuls of baby spinach leaves
freshly ground black pepper

Tortillas are a good source of fibre, which helps with digestion. Cream cheese provides calcium, which helps to strengthen bones, and spinach leaves are a good source of folic acid, which helps to prevent birth defects in early pregnancy.

1 Spread the flour tortillas with the cream cheese. Cover with the tomatoes, red pepper, and spinach leaves, and wrap up.

2 If you fancy them warm, wrap in foil and put into a hot oven for 5–10 minutes. Otherwise, eat them as they are.

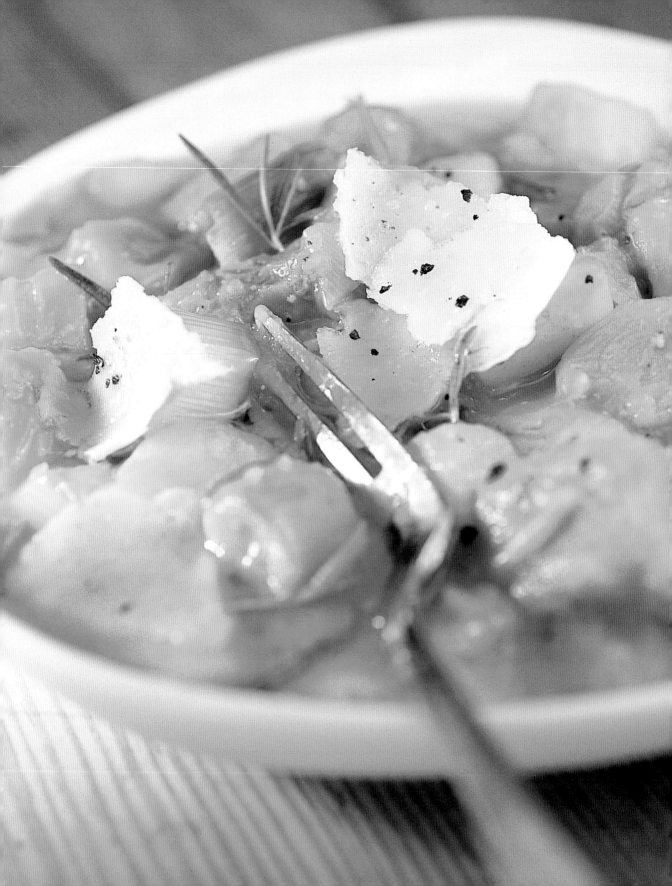

vegetarian pregnancy
dinners

root vegetable stew

makes: 4 portions

storage: up to 2–3 days in the refrigerator or up to 3 months in the freezer

2 medium butternut squash
1 litre (1¾ pints) vegetable stock
1 small onion, peeled and halved
1 bay leaf
salt and black pepper, to taste
2 sprigs fresh rosemary
40g (1½oz) butter
2 medium leeks into 2.5cm (1 inch) pieces
2 cloves garlic, peeled and sliced
2 small parsnips, peeled and cut into bite-size pieces
2 x 400g tins butter beans, drained and rinsed
grated vegetarian Parmesan-style cheese, to serve
garlic bread, to serve

This is based on a dish served in the renowned Irish vegetarian restaurant Café Paradiso in Cork – a truly inspirational place.

1 Peel and deseed the squash and chop into bite-size pieces. Put half the squash into a saucepan with the stock, onion, bay leaf, salt, pepper and 1 rosemary sprig. Bring to the boil and simmer gently for 30 minutes.

2 Remove the onion, bay leaf, and rosemary. Purée the cooked squash and the remaining liquid until smooth. Heat the butter in a large casserole dish and sauté the leeks and garlic gently for 5 minutes, until the leeks are just beginning to soften.

3 Add the remaining squash and the parsnips, and continue to cook gently for 5 minutes, then add the remaining sprig of rosemary and season. Add the butter beans and the puréed squash. Bring to the boil and simmer gently for 25–30 minutes or longer until the squash and parsnips are tender. Leave to cool completely. Pour into freezer-proof containers and freeze.

4 Serve with the Parmesan-style cheese (or any other vegetarian hard cheese) sprinkled over the top and garlic bread to mop up the juices.

penne with tomato sauce

makes: 4 portions

storage: up to 2–3 days in the refrigerator

250g (9oz) penne
250g (9oz) sunblush tomatoes
1 clove garlic, peeled and chopped
1 shallot, peeled and chopped
sea salt and ground black pepper, to taste
2 tsp aged balsamic vinegar
2 tbsp extra virgin olive oil, plus extra for drizzling
6 basil leaves, torn
200g (7oz) rocket leaves, to serve

Serve this pasta dish with a fresh green salad. Pasta is a great complex carbohydrate, which provides slow-release energy to the body. Sunblush tomatoes contain betacarotene and vitamin C, both of which help to boost the immune system.

1 Bring a pan of water to the boil. Add the pasta, and cook according to the instructions on the pack.

2 Blitz the remaining ingredients, except the basil and rocket, in a food processor for a few seconds, until the mixture resembles a chunky salsa. Mix with the cooked pasta.

3 Drizzle with a little extra olive oil and sprinkle with the basil. Serve hot or cold with the rocket leaves or any other green salad.

squash and thyme tarts

makes: 6 portions

storage: up to 2–3 days in the refrigerator

for the pastry:
180g (6¼oz) plain flour
pinch of salt
1 tsp finely chopped fresh thyme
90g (3½oz) chilled unsalted butter, cut into small pieces
1 large free-range egg (optional)
ice-cold water

for the filling:
180g (1lb) squash, halved and deseeded
1 tbsp olive oil
25g (1oz) butter
1 small leek, chopped
2 cloves garlic, peeled and chopped
1 large free-range egg
40g (1½oz) vegetarian Parmesan-style cheese, grated
90ml 3fl oz) double cream
45ml (1½fl oz) full-fat milk
fresh thyme, plus extra sprigs to serve

for the relish:
25g (1oz) butter
2 red onions, peeled and finely chopped
1 medium beetroot, cooked, peeled, and finely chopped
1 tbsp balsamic vinegar

This makes a perfect supper served with a fresh watercress salad. It isn't necessary to add egg to the pastry recipe; you can either use 1 free-range egg and approximately 2 tbsp cold water, or just 3–4 tbsp cold water.

1 Preheat the oven to 200°C/400°F/gas mark 6. Roast the squash for 40 minutes, until soft. Set aside

2 Make the pastry: sift the flour and salt into a food processor, add the thyme, and pulse for a few seconds. Add the butter and process to make fine breadcrumbs. Keeping the machine running, add the egg (if using) and a little water, if necessary, 1 tbsp at a time. If the pastry is still in crumbly pieces, add a little more water. Alternatively, to make by hand, sift the flour into a large bowl with the salt. Add the chopped butter and rub the fat into the flour. Stir in the thyme. Add the egg (if using) and gradually pour in enough water to bring the mixture together to form a ball. Wrap in cling film and chill for at least 30 minutes.

3 Roll out the pastry and line four 10cm (4in) tart tins. Chill for 30 minutes.

4 Lower the oven to 180°C/350°F/gas mark 4. Heat a baking sheet until hot. Cover the pastry with sheets of baking paper and baking beans, place the tins on the sheet, and bake for 10 minutes. Remove the paper and beans, and cook for another 5 minutes.

5 Meanwhile, caramelize the red onions for the relish by melting the butter in a frying pan and gently sautéing the onions, uncovered, for 30-40 minutes, stirring often until they are meltingly soft and have reduced and taken on a glazed appearance.

6 Heat the oil and butter in a small saucepan, add the leek and garlic, and sauté for a few minutes, until soft. Scoop out the cooked squash flesh and put in a food processor with the egg, 30g (1oz) Parmesan-style cheese, cream, milk, and thyme. Process until smooth (or mix well by hand).

7 Fill the tart cases with the squash mixture, then top with the remaining cheese. Bake for about 20 minutes, until slightly puffed and golden.

8 Mix together the ingredients for the beetroot and red onion relish and serve with the tarts.

Thai-style curry with tofu

makes: 4 portions

storage: best eaten immediately, or up to 2 days in the refrigerator

25ml (1fl oz) sesame oil
2 red onions, peeled and sliced
3 cloves garlic, peeled and chopped
2 red chillies, deseeded and finely sliced (with a few seeds for a little kick), plus a little chilli powder
4cm (1½in) piece of fresh ginger, peeled and finely chopped
2 tbsp tomato purée
1 stalk lemon grass
grated zest of 1 unwaxed lime
400g (14oz) soft tofu, chopped
200g (7oz) sugar snap peas, sliced
300ml (10½fl oz) coconut milk
200ml (7fl oz) vegetable stock
2–3 tsp lime juice
3–4 large handfuls of baby spinach leaves
large handful of coriander leaves, chopped
large handful of cashew nuts, chopped and toasted, or sesame seeds or pumpkin seeds, toasted

Tofu is the Japanese name given to soybean curd and is a very good vegetarian source of protein, calcium, and iron, which is essential for a developing foetus. It has the added advantage of being low in saturated fat, contains no cholesterol, and has almost no sodium. Spinach is a good source of folic acid, betacarotene, and iron. Coconut milk also provides some calcium, aiding in the development of strong teeth and bones. Ginger is thought to be very good for relieving morning sickness. (Do not eat nuts if there is any family history of allergies.)

1   Heat the oil in a frying pan or wok. Add the onions and fry, stirring well, until deeply coloured. Add the garlic, chillies, and ginger, and fry for another minute, stirring all the time.

2   Add the tomato purée, lemon grass (crushed with a rolling pin), lime zest, tofu, and sugar snap peas, and stir gently over a medium heat for a minute, to coat the tofu.

3   Add the coconut milk, stock, and lime juice, and simmer uncovered for 4 minutes. Add the spinach and toss together. Cook for another 2 minutes.

4   Serve with lots of fresh coriander and cashew nuts or seeds scattered over the top.

stuffed orange peppers

makes: 4 portions

storage: up to 2–3 days in the refrigerator

2 orange and 2 yellow peppers
75g (2½oz) brioche crumbs
2 tbsp pine nuts, toasted and roughly chopped
handful each of flat-leaf parsley and mint, chopped
250g (9oz) vegetarian haloumi, grated
handful of black olives, pitted and chopped (optional)
grated zest of 1 unwaxed orange
2 tbsp extra virgin olive oil
sea salt and freshly ground black pepper, to taste

Brioche is a sweet, rich bread ideal for stuffing roasted peppers. Haloumi is a very good source of protein and calcium. Peppers are an excellent source of vitamin C. Pine nuts are a good source of magnesium and zinc, which are important for growth. (Do not eat nuts if there is any history of allergies.)

1   Preheat the oven to 190°C/ 375°F/gas mark 5. Put the whole peppers in a roasting tin and roast for 45 minutes, until soft.

2   Put the brioche crumbs on to a baking sheet and toast in the oven for 5 minutes, turning the crumbs now and then until golden and crisp. Transfer to a bowl.

3   Add the pine nuts, herbs, cheese, olives, orange zest, and half the oil to the crumbs, mix together, and season to taste.

4   Remove the stalks from the peppers and scoop out the seeds. Fill the peppers with the crumb mixture and drizzle over the remaining oil. Bake for 15 minutes, until warmed through.

squash and cumin soup

Butternut squash is very high in betacarotene, which is essential for growth and a healthy immune system.

makes: 6 portions

storage: soup lasts up to 2–3 days in the refrigerator, or up to 3 months in the freezer

1 tbsp olive oil
1 large onion, peeled and finely
  chopped
2 medium cloves garlic, peeled and
  chopped
½ tsp cumin seeds
½ tsp ground cumin
1kg (2lb 3oz) butternut squash,
  peeled and cubed
1.1 litres (38fl oz) vegetable stock
1 tbsp tomato purée
freshly ground black pepper, to
  taste
a little semi-skimmed milk
  (optional)

1 Heat the oil in a saucepan and sweat the onion until soft. Add the garlic, cumin seeds, and ground cumin, and cook for another minute.

2 Mix in the butternut squash, add the stock and tomato purée, and bring to the boil. Cover with a lid and simmer for 30 minutes, until the squash is very soft.

3 Using a hand blender, purée the soup until smooth. Season with black pepper. If the mixture is too thick, thin it with some semi-skimmed milk.

4 If freezing, leave to cool completely. Pour into freezer-proof containers and freeze. Thaw completely before heating through in a saucepan.

sweet potato frittata

Sweet potatoes are a very good source of betacarotene, which helps to boost the immune system. Spinach is a very good source of iron and folic acid, while eggs provide protein.

makes: 2 portions

storage: best eaten immediately, or up to 2 days in the refrigerator

150g (5½oz) sweet potatoes, peeled
  and chopped into small pieces
50g (1¾oz) fresh leaf spinach
75g (2½oz) fresh or frozen peas
2 tbsp olive oil
½ large onion, peeled and finely
  chopped
4 large free-range eggs
freshly ground black pepper, to
  taste

1 Bring a pan of water to the boil, add the sweet potatoes, and cook for about 10–15 minutes until tender. Drain and whizz in a food processor or blender until puréed.

2 Heat a little water in a pan and add the spinach and peas. Cook for 1–2 minutes, until the spinach has wilted, then drain.

3 Heat half the oil in a small frying pan and sauté the onion until soft.

4 In a bowl, whisk the eggs, then add the onion, puréed sweet potato, spinach, and peas. Give the mixture a quick stir without totally blending everything together. Season with a little freshly ground black pepper.

5 Heat the rest of the oil in a small frying pan over a medium heat. Turn the heat down and pour the egg mixture into the pan. Leave to cook until the egg is almost set (about 5 minutes).

6 Preheat the grill to high and finish cooking the frittata under the grill. Serve in wedges.

Moroccan spiced lentil soup

makes: 4 portions

storage: soup lasts up to 2–3 days in the refrigerator, or up to 3 months in the freezer

2 tbsp olive oil
5 carrots, peeled and chopped
2 celery sticks, chopped
2 onions, peeled and chopped
5 cloves garlic, peeled and chopped
1 tsp each ground cinnamon, allspice, and cumin
150g (5½oz) green lentils
400g (14oz) tin chopped tomatoes
200ml (7fl oz) fruity red wine
2 litres (3½ pints) vegetable stock
14 pieces mixed prunes and apricots
handful each of fresh flat-leaf parsley and mint, chopped
natural Greek yogurt and crusty bread, to serve (optional)

Lentils provide protein, which helps with growth and development. Prunes and apricots provide fibre, which aids the digestion process.

1 Heat the oil in a large saucepan and sauté the carrot, celery, and onions for about 5 minutes. Add the garlic and sauté for another 5 minutes, until the vegetables begin to soften.

2 Add the spices and stir to coat the vegetables, releasing their aroma.

3 Add the lentils, tomatoes, red wine, and stock. Bring to the boil and simmer, uncovered, for about 40 minutes, by which time the lentils should be completely cooked through.

4 Add the fruit and gently cook for another 10 minutes. Roughly purée in a food processor or blender, and stir in the herbs. If you like, serve it with a dollop of natural Greek yogurt on top and fresh, crusty bread.

quick vegetable stir-fry

makes: 2 portions

storage: best eaten immediately, or up to 2 days in the refrigerator

2 tbsp olive oil
4 tsp sesame oil
2 cloves garlic, peeled and crushed
about 15g (½oz) fresh ginger, peeled and very finely chopped
250g (9oz) tofu, cut into cubes
2 spring onions, finely sliced diagonally
1 red pepper, deseeded and thinly sliced
200g (7oz) baby corn, sliced in half
200g (7oz) mange-tout, halved lengthways
100g (3¾oz) bean sprouts
25g (1oz) cashew nuts, toasted
2 tsp light soy sauce
freshly ground black pepper
200g (7oz) cooked egg noodles (optional)
2 tbsp toasted sesame seeds

Tofu is bland, so you need to mix it with other ingredients, such as a simple marinade, to give it flavour. Stir-fried vegetables are great, because they are cooked so quickly that they retain most of their nutritional value, and you can add any fresh vegetables that you have to hand. (Do not eat seeds or their products if there is any family history of allergies.)

1 Put half of each of the oils into a small bowl, add half the garlic and half the ginger, and mix together. Add the tofu, cover, and leave to marinate for at least 30 minutes.

2 Heat a wok and add the tofu in its marinade. Stir-fry gently for a few minutes, then transfer to a plate.

3 Put the remaining oil into the wok and heat over a high heat. Add the remaining garlic and ginger, and the spring onions, and stir-fry for 1 minute.

4 Cook the hardest vegetables first. First add the pepper and baby corn, and stir-fry for 1 minute. Add the mange-tout and cook for 1 minute more, then add the bean sprouts and cashew nuts. Cook for another minute, stirring constantly.

5 Add the soy sauce and season to taste with black pepper. As soon as the vegetables are cooked, but still crunchy, add the noodles (if using) and the tofu, and stir-fy for a minute. Sprinkle over the sesame seeds and serve.

macaroni cheese with onions

makes: 4 portions

storage: up to 2 days in the refrigerator or up to 3 months in the freezer

60g (2oz) unsalted butter
1 tbsp olive oil
3 large red onions, peeled and sliced
50g (1¾oz) plain flour
600ml (21fl oz) full-fat milk
200g (7oz) medium or mature vegetarian Cheddar, grated
salt and black pepper, to taste
300g (10½oz) macaroni

Pasta is a great source of complex carbohydrates, providing both resistant starch, which is broken down slowly in the body to boost energy reserves, and fibre, which helps to maintain a healthy digestive tract. The sweet caramelized onions make a welcome addition to this otherwise classic comfort dish.

1 Preheat the oven to 180°C/350°F/gas mark 4. Melt 10g (¼oz) of the unsalted butter with the oil in a heavy-based frying pan. Add the onion and cook, stirring frequently, until soft and slightly caramelized – about 10 minutes.

2 Put the remaining butter in a small pan and melt over a gentle heat. Add the flour and cook for 1 minute, stirring constantly with a wooden spoon to make a smooth, glossy paste.

3 Take the pan off the heat and add a little milk, stirring continuously with a wooden spoon until the milk is completely combined. Gradually add the rest of the milk, still stirring constantly, to get a smooth sauce.

4 Return the pan to a low heat and cook the sauce gently for 5–6 minutes, stirring constantly. Add three-quarters of the cheese, taste and season.

5 Cook the macaroni until *al dente* – it should still have a little bite. Drain.

6 Mix the macaroni and onion together in an ovenproof dish, then pour over the cheese sauce. Sprinkle with the remaining cheese and bake for 15–20 minutes, or until golden and the sauce is bubbling around the edges.

7 Alternatively, the macaroni cheese can be frozen before it is cooked in the oven. Leave the prepared dish to cool, then wrap in foil and freeze. Thaw thoroughly before cooking at 180°C/350°F/gas mark 4 for 20–25 minutes.

spinach and ricotta tart

makes: 6 portions

storage: up to 2–3 days in the refrigerator

50g (1¾oz) walnuts, toasted and roughly chopped
375g (13oz) ready-rolled puff pastry
large knob of butter
1 tbsp olive oil
3 large red onions, peeled and finely sliced
2 tbsp light soft brown sugar
200g (7oz) fresh baby leaf spinach
125g (4½oz) vegetarian mascarpone
200ml (7fl oz) double cream (or ½ double cream and ½ full-fat milk)
3 large free-range eggs
freshly ground black pepper
grating of fresh nutmeg
300g (10½oz) vegetarian ricotta

As well as providing iron, spinach is also a good source of folic acid, which is essential during pregnancy. It also contains vitamins C and E, both of which are antioxidants that protect against heart disease and strokes. (Do not eat nuts if there is any family history of allergies.)

1 Preheat the oven 150°C/300°F/gas mark 2. Scatter the walnuts over the pastry sheet, fold over the pastry, then roll out again into a circle large enough to line a 20cm (8 inch) tart tin. Gently ease the pastry into the tin, prick the base all over with a fork, cover, and chill for 30 minutes.

2 Bake blind for 15 minutes, lined with baking parchment and beans or rice, then remove the paper and beans or rice, and bake for another 5 minutes.

3 Heat the butter and oil in a heavy-based frying pan and sauté the onions for at least 10–15 minutes, or until soft. Add the sugar and continue to cook, stirring frequently, for a further 5 minutes, or until sticky and caramelized.

4 Steam the spinach for a few minutes until the leaves have just wilted, squeeze out the water, then chop into small pieces.

5 Whisk together the mascarpone, cream, and eggs, then season with the pepper and nutmeg. Add the ricotta and gently mix together.

6 Scatter the spinach and onion over the tart base, then pour in the cheese filling. Bake for 45–50 minutes, or until set, well risen, and golden.

mushroom and tarragon stew

makes: 4 portions

storage: best eaten immediately, or up to 1–2 days in the refrigerator. (Rice should not be reheated, but can be served cold)

25g (1oz) dried porcini mushrooms
250ml (9fl oz) boiling water
3 tbsp olive oil
2 onions, peeled and chopped
2–3 cloves garlic, peeled and crushed
700g (1lb 9oz) field or chestnut mushrooms, washed and chopped into bite-size pieces
1 tbsp marsala (optional)
1 tbsp tamari or soy sauce
400g tin chopped tomatoes
large handful of fresh tarragon, chopped
4 tbsp sour cream
rice, or mashed potato, to serve

Mushrooms provide copper, which helps the body to absorb iron, potassium, which helps to regulate blood pressure, and phosphorus, vital for healthy teeth and bones.

1 Put the porcini mushrooms in a jug and pour over the boiling water. Leave to soak for at least 30 minutes. Lift out the mushrooms with a slotted spoon, squeeze out the liquid and reserve. Finely chop the mushrooms. Strain the liquid through kitchen paper to remove any grit and reserve the liquid.

2 Heat the oil in a large heavy-based pan and sauté the onions gently for 10 minutes until soft. Add the garlic and cook for another couple of minutes. Add the mushrooms and fry for 5 minutes, until slightly soft and golden.

3 Add the marsala (if using) or 1 tbsp of the porcini stock and cook for 1 minute.

4 Cover and cook for a further 5 minutes. Add the remaining porcini stock, tamari, tomatoes, and most of the tarragon. Cover and simmer gently for 15 minutes.

5 Spoon the stew on to 4 plates. Top each with a dollop of sour cream and sprinkle over a little extra tarragon.

spicy couscous with roasted veg

makes: 6 portions

storage: up to 2–3 days in the refrigerator

2 each red and yellow peppers, deseeded
2 medium aubergines
8 ripe tomatoes, halved
6 cloves garlic, peeled
2 red onions, peeled and sliced into thin wedges
2 tbsp olive oil
sea salt and freshly ground black pepper, to taste
500g (1lb 2oz) couscous
750ml (26½fl oz) boiling vegetable stock (or enough to cover couscous)
large knob of butter
1 tsp crushed dried red chilli
2–3 tsp harissa paste

Couscous is a complex carbohydrate, which is important for providing energy to the body. Peppers, tomatoes, and aubergines are all sources of vitamin C, which provides natural immunity.

1 Preheat the oven to 200°C/ 400°F/gas mark 6. Cut the peppers into chunks and slice the aubergines. Arrange all the vegetables in a roasting tin, pour over the oil, and toss around until coated. Season and roast in the oven for 35–45 minutes, turning once, until cooked and golden at the edges.

2 Put the couscous into an ovenproof dish, cover the grains with boiling stock, and leave for 10 minutes for the grains to swell.

3 Dot the butter over the top, season, and sprinkle with the chilli. Cover with foil and bake alongside the vegetables for 25 minutes.

4 Mix the couscous, vegetables, and harissa together and serve.

lentils with feta and mint salsa

makes: 4 portions

storage: best eaten immediately, or up to 2–3 days in the refrigerator

350g Puy lentils
4 red peppers
2 tbsp olive oil
3 red onions, peeled and sliced
a pinch of salt
1 tbsp balsamic vinegar
1 tsp soft brown sugar
handfuls of baby salad leaves
a little olive oil and red wine vinegar
handful of mint, leaves chopped
250g (9oz) vegetarian feta

for the salsa:
3 garlic cloves, peeled
1 medium red chilli, deseeded
handful of flat-leaf parsley
handful of mint leaves
1 tsp Dijon mustard
2 tsp red wine vinegar
4 tbsp olive oil

Lentils are a good source of protein, but they are particularly good when eaten with rice, bread, or other cereal products to help provide you with all the essential amino acids for growth and development. Ideally, try to eat this salad with a fresh bread roll.

1 Preheat the oven to 200°C/400°F/gas mark 6. Rinse the lentils, place in a saucepan, and cover generously with cold water. Bring to the boil and simmer for 15–20 minutes until cooked. (They may need longer if not fresh.)

2 Roast the red peppers in the oven until the skin has blackened and blistered. Pop into a plastic bag and, when cool enough, peel. Cut into thin strips.

3 Heat the oil and sauté the onions with a good pinch of salt until softened and beginning to caramelize. Add the vinegar and sugar, and cook for a further 5 minutes, stirring frequently.

4 To make the salsa, throw all the ingredients except the oil into a food processor and pulse to a coarse paste. Stir in the oil and season well.

5 Dress the salad leaves with a little oil and vinegar. Mix the caramelized onion and mint through the lentils and pile on top of the salad leaves. Top with crumbled feta and red pepper strips, and finish with a spoonful of the salsa. Serve with bread rolls.

vegetarian shepherd's pie

makes: 4 portions

storage: up to 2 days in the refrigerator or up to 3 months in the freezer

a little butter
2 tbsp olive oil
1 onion, peeled and finely chopped
2 cloves garlic, peeled and crushed
2 carrots, peeled and chopped
400g (14oz) swede, peeled and chopped
3–4 sprigs of thyme, finely chopped
2 sprigs of rosemary, finely chopped
75g (2½oz) split red lentils
75g (2½oz) green lentils
300g tinned cannellini beans, rinsed and drained
300g tinned black-eyed peas, rinsed and drained
750ml (26½fl oz) boiling vegetable stock
200g (7oz) cherry tomatoes, chopped
handful of fresh basil leaves, torn

for the mash top:
900g (2lb) potatoes, peeled and chopped
200g (7oz) vegetarian mozzarella ball, shredded
large knob of butter
2 tbsp milk
30g (1oz) vegetarian Parmesan-style cheese, finely grated

If you want to make this dish in advance, you will need to cook it for slightly longer than 20 minutes in the oven: it is more likely to need 30–40 minutes.

1 Butter a large ovenproof dish. Heat 1 tbsp of the oil in large heavy-based saucepan. Sauté the onion gently for 10 minutes until soft. Add half the garlic and sweat for a few more minutes. Add the carrot and swede, and sauté for a further 10 minutes.

2 Add the thyme, rosemary, lentils, beans, and black-eyed peas and stir until well combined. Add the stock, bring up to a simmer, and cook for 20 minutes, or until the lentils are soft. Spoon into the ovenproof dish.

3 Heat the remaining oil in the pan, add the remaining garlic and the tomatoes and basil, and sauté for a few minutes.

4 Preheat the oven to 180°C/350°F/gas mark 4. Meanwhile, bring a pan of water to the boil and cook the potatoes for 15 minutes or until tender. Drain and return to the pan. Over a gentle heat, add the mozzarella cheese, butter, and milk, and mash until smooth.

5 Spread the potato mixture over the beans, sprinkle with the cheese and bake for 20–25 minutes or until the top is golden.

6 Alternatively, the shepherd's pie can be frozen before it is cooked in the oven. Leave the prepared pie to cool, then wrap in foil and freeze. Thaw thoroughly before cooking as above.

vanilla roasted fruit

makes: 4 portions

storage: up to 2–3 days in the refrigerator

900g (2lb) plums, halved and stoned
3 peaches or nectarines, halved and stoned
1 vanilla pod
1–2 tbsp golden caster sugar, to taste

Choose any fruit in season: plums, nectarines, figs, cherries, pears, and apples all work really well.

1 Preheat the oven to 200°C/400°F/gas mark 6. Put the plums and nectarines into an ovenproof dish.

2 Cut a slit in the vanilla pod and scrape half the seeds into a bowl. Add the sugar, and mix together. Scatter the vanilla sugar over the fruit and roast for approximately 10 minutes, until the fruit is slightly soft, but still holding its shape. Alternatively, put the fruit under a hot grill for 5 minutes.

3 Serve with yogurt and cereal, or use as the base for a crumble.

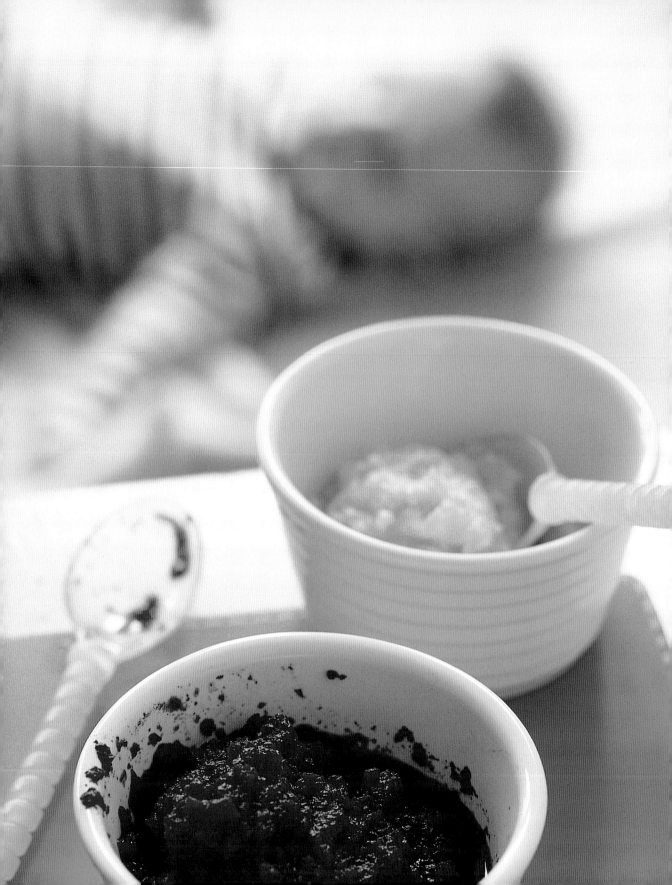

When your baby is 7 months old, you may find that she is ready to progress from soft purées quite quickly to 'mushy' fruits and vegetables with a slightly thicker texture, and that your baby wants to feed herself quite early in the weaning process. If so, you could introduce her to soft finger foods such as pieces of banana, avocado, mango, or peas. If she is able to pass food from hand to mouth, most experts believe that she will also be able to chew and swallow soft foods – with or without teeth.

Try to feed her fruits or vegetables that you are cooking for the rest of the family. For example, when you are cooking vegetables, such as potatoes for your family, cook the potatoes (without any salt), then take some out for your baby and mash. Alternatively, cook a few portions of puréed fruits or vegetables for your baby and freeze.

The amount of portions each recipe serves is only intended as a guide; the amount your baby eats will depend on a number of factors, including her appetite, her weight, and her age.

baby
recipes

vegetable
purées

Some parents like to start their baby off on single-food purées. This is a great way to introduce your baby to a variety of tastes. You may need to add breast milk, formula milk, or baby rice to these purées to create the desired consistency. You could also try giving your baby some of the softer fruits and vegetables as finger foods, once she has been weaning for six weeks or when your baby is seven months, whichever is later. If you are feeding a baby pieces of vegetables, make sure they are not so small that your baby is at risk of choking.

asparagus – steamed spears or puréed

Asparagus is great for the immune system and is a good source of betacarotene, essential for healthy skin and lungs. It also contains vitamin C, potassium, folic acid, and riboflavin. Use fresh asparagus (look for stalks with clean, pale-green ends) and choose medium-size stalks. Asparagus is best eaten on the day it is bought. Snap off the tough ends of the stalks. Cut each stalk into four pieces and steam for 5–10 minutes, then whizz with a hand-held blender (or in a food processor or blender) until smooth, with no stringy bits.

beetroot – puréed

Beetroot is a good source of vitamins and minerals, especially vitamins B_6 and C, betacarotene, potassium, calcium, iron, and folic acid. It is a great immune-boosting food. Cut off the stalk ends of the beetroot. Boil for 25–30 minutes, until tender. Drain and leave to cool, then peel. Whizz the flesh with a hand-held blender (or in a food processor or blender) until smooth.

avocado – puréed or large pieces

Avocados are rich in monounsaturated fats, which promote healthy skin. They are also easily digested, making them great for babies. Avocados can be served raw: pick a ripe one that gives slightly when pressed around the neck. Cut the avocado in half, then twist to separate. Scrape the flesh from one half into a bowl. Whizz in a blender. Make this just before serving.

peas – puréed

Peas are rich in vitamin C, the B vitamins, and iron. Put frozen peas in a pan of boiling water, bring back to the boil and cook for 1 minute. Drain. Whizz with a hand-held blender (or in a food processor or blender) until smooth or, for just-weaned babies, push through a sieve. Fresh peas should be cooked for longer, puréed, and sieved for babies up to seven months.

broccoli – puréed or steamed florets

Broccoli is an excellent source of iron, particularly because it is a good source of vitamin C, essential in aiding the absorption of iron. It is also an immune-boosting food. Cut off the hard stalk from the broccoli head. Remove a quarter of the florets and steam them for 5–10 minutes until tender. Whizz with a hand-held blender (or in a food processor or blender) until smooth.

cauliflower – puréed or steamed florets

Cauliflower has high levels of vitamin C and folic acid. Try adding some tender green inner leaves to the purée, as this will increase its vitamin C content. Put the cauliflower florets and tender leaves into a steamer and steam for 10 minutes (or boil for 8 minutes), until tender. Whizz with a hand-held blender (or in a food processor or blender) until smooth.

carrot – puréed or steamed pieces

Carrots are an excellent first food for babies because they rarely trigger an allergic reaction. Smaller carrots may be sweeter, but older, darker carrots have a higher nutrient content. Carrots are also a good treatment for diarrhoea. If you buy organic carrots there is no need to peel them; just scrub them well. Non-organic carrots will need to be peeled. Chop your carrot into small pieces and boil or steam until tender (approximately 5 minutes). Whizz with a hand-held blender (or in a food processor or blender) until smooth.

parsnip – puréed or steamed pieces

Parsnips are a good source of minerals and vitamins. They also help to relieve constipation. Peel the parsnip and cut it into small pieces, then steam over boiling water for 6–8 minutes, until tender. Whizz with a hand-held blender (or in a food processor or blender) until smooth.

courgette – puréed or steamed pieces

Courgettes are rich in vitamin C, folic acid, and potassium. Choose small, young courgettes, which will not need to be peeled, as they have tender, soft skins. It is better to choose organic, as any pesticide residues would be found in the skin. Remove the ends from the courgettes and slice into small rounds. Steam or boil until tender (10–15 minutes). Whizz with a hand-held blender (or in a food processor or blender) until smooth, with no stringy bits.

fruit
purées

You may need to add breast milk, formula milk, or baby rice to these purées to create the desired consistency. You can serve them smooth for newly weaned babies or slightly chunky after six weeks of weaning when your baby is seven months, whichever is later. All fruits except for banana should be cooked at the beginning of weaning. If you are feeding a baby pieces of fruit, make sure they are not so small that your baby is at risk of choking.

mango – pieces or purée
Mango is naturally sweet and easy to digest. Rich in vitamin C, minerals, and antioxidants, it is great for the immune system and for convalescing babies. Choose ripe mangoes; unripe ones can cause stomach upsets. Peel the fruit, then wash the peeling knife before chopping. Slice the mango down each side of the stone. Scoop out the flesh using a spoon (if you can't do this the fruit is probably not ripe enough). Steam or simmer in 2–3 tbsp water for a few minutes, until soft. Whizz with a hand-held blender (or in a food processor or blender).

apple – puréed or steamed pieces
When cooked, apples' sweet, soft purée is always popular with babies. Apples are rich in antioxidants, so they are a good immune-boosting food. They are also good for diarrhoea and constipation. Try to buy organic, tree-ripened apples. Peel and core the apple. Cut it into small pieces and simmer in water or steam for 5 minutes, until soft. Whizz with a hand-held blender (or in a food processor or blender).

You can also bake apples. Cut the fruit in half and scoop out the core. Score a line around its middle and bake at 180°C/350°F/ gas mark 4 for 25 minutes, until soft. Scoop the flesh from the skin and whizz with a hand-held blender.

banana – pieces or purée
Bananas are a great first food, but the purée can be a bit thick for a baby to swallow, so add a little boiled water or breast milk or formula milk. Buy really ripe fruit, as the starch will have turned to sugar, making it easier on a baby's delicate digestive system. Bananas are also good for diarrhoea and constipation. Peel your banana and mash or purée. Dilute it with water or breast milk or formula milk as necessary. Alternatively, bake a banana in its skin for 20 minutes at 180°C/350°F/gas mark 4. Cool and peel, then mash the flesh thoroughly, making sure there are no lumps.

blueberry – purée

Blueberries can be hard for babies to digest, so they are best puréed and sieved or put through a Mouli until weaning has been underway for at least 4 months. Blueberries have natural antibacterial properties, which help to prevent mild colds, and they are also excellent for treating diarrhoea. Put the blueberries in a saucepan with a little water and simmer gently until the fruit bursts open. Whizz with a hand-held blender (or in a food processor or blender) until smooth.

cherry – halved and stones removed or purée

Cherries have good cleansing and antioxidant properties, which make them great for building up resistance. They are also good for constipation. They have high levels of vitamin C, potassium, and magnesium. Halve and stone your cherries, then cook them in a small pan with a little water. Once soft, allow to cool, then whizz with a hand-held blender (or in a food processor or blender).

apricot – pieces or purée

Apricots are rich in betacarotene, which the body converts into vitamin A. They are good for constipation – especially dried apricots, but these are best given to babies more than nine months old. Apricots also have high levels of iron and potassium. First skin your fruit by putting it in boiling water. Leave for 1 minute, then slip the skin off using a sharp knife. Remove the stones, finely chop and cook the flesh with 1 tbsp water until soft. Whizz with a hand-held blender (or in a food processor or blender).

melon – pieces or purée

Cantaloupe, Galia, and Charentais are the sweetest varieties. Melons are good for digestion, but are also a mild laxative. Peel your melon and remove the seeds. Simmer the melon with a little water for a few minutes, until soft. When buying melon, choose ones that feel heavy for their size and have a sweet aroma. Whizz with a hand-held blender (or in a food processor or blender).

pear – pieces or purée

Pears are a great first food because they have a fairly neutral flavour. They relieve constipation and are good for convalescence. Peel and core your pear, and cut into bite-size pieces. Cook gently in a small pan with a little water until soft. Whizz with a hand-held blender (or in a food processor or blender).

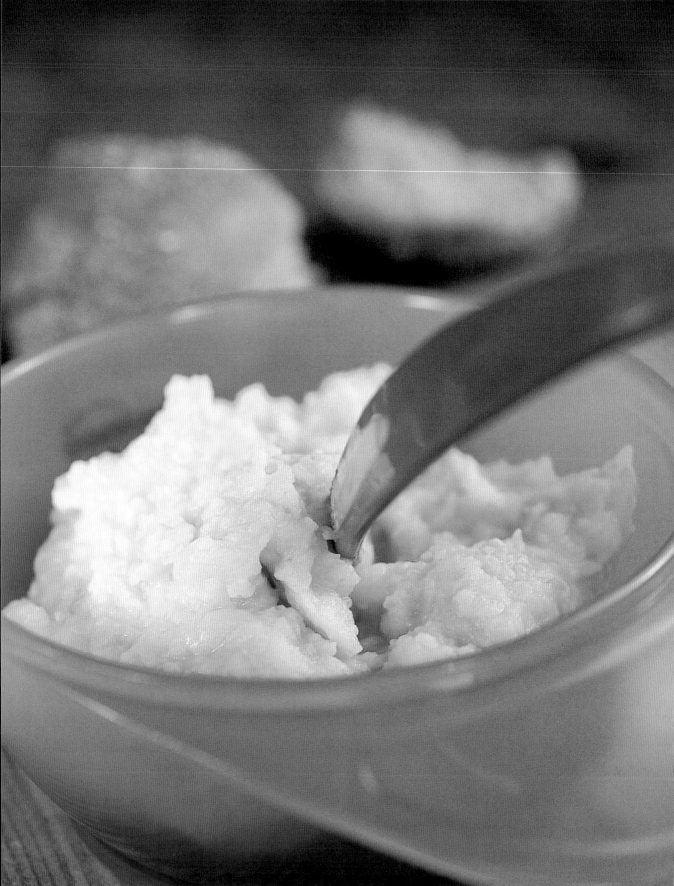

vegetarian savouries
7–9 months

puréed orange lentils and carrot

suitable from 9 months

makes: 6 baby portions and 2 adult portions for a soup base

storage: up to 24 hours in the refrigerator or up to 2 months in the freezer

1 tbsp olive oil
1 small onion, peeled and finely chopped
2 large carrots, peeled and cut into small chunks
2 medium potatoes, peeled and cut into small chunks
75g (2½oz) split red lentils
2 dried apricots, chopped
750ml (26fl oz) water
soft bread, to serve

Once your baby reaches 7 months it is an ideal time to start to introduce some protein such as lentils into his diet. It is sensible to mix the lentils with familiar vegetables such as carrots and potatoes, as this will help him adjust to the new flavour and help with digestion. The dried apricots add some iron to this purée, too.

1   Heat the oil in a saucepan and fry the onion for 3–4 minutes or until soft.
2   Add the carrot and potato and fry for 10 minutes or until tender.
3   Add the lentils and apricots and stir well. Pour over the water and cook for 25 minutes or until the lentils are cooked and the vegetables tender.
4   Purée with a hand-held blender (or in a food processor or blender) until completely smooth. If the purée is too thick, let it down with a little warm water or breast milk or formula milk.
5   If freezing, leave to cool completely. Pour into freezer-proof containers and freeze. Thaw completely before heating through in a saucepan.

leek, carrot and tofu purée

makes: 5–6 portions

storage: up to 3–4 days in the refrigerator

1 large leek, washed and chopped
2 large carrots, peeled and chopped
50g (1¾oz) silken tofu

Leek is a member of the onion family and has a similar flavour to an onion, but it is much milder. It is an ideal vegetable to give to babies to help get them used to a new flavour, without it being too overpowering. Silken tofu is an easy way of adding some protein to your baby's diet.

1   Bring a pan of water to the boil and steam or boil the vegetables until just tender. Drain.
2   Add to the tofu and whizz with a hand-held blender (or in a food processor or blender) until you have the desired consistency.

tomato and butter bean paté

suitable from 7 months

makes: 3–4 baby portions and 1–2 adult portions

storage: up to 2–3 days in the refrigerator

4 ripe plum tomatoes
400g tin butter beans,
  drained and rinsed
3 tbsp olive oil
1 clove garlic, peeled and crushed
  (optional)
1 tbsp lemon juice
2 tbsp finely chopped fresh flat-leaf
  parsley or coriander leaves
freshly ground black pepper
fingers of toast or pitta bread,
  to serve (if your baby is confident
  with chewing)

The main reason for making this paté, other than the fact that it is a simple and easy way to feed your baby beans, is because it tastes so good it is the prefect lunch for you as well. I think it is important to encourage your baby to try new flavours such as garlic and herbs when she is still quite young, to show that food can be really varied and exciting.

1 Put the tomatoes in a bowl, cover with boiling water and leave for 2 minutes. Drain and rinse with cold water. Remove the skins and roughly chop the tomatoes. Add to the other ingredients except the toast.

2 Whizz all the ingredients together with a hand-held blender (or in a food processor or blender) to a smooth purée. Season to taste with freshly ground black pepper. If it's a little too thick, thin with some tomato passata. Serve with toast or pitta bread fingers.

avocado and cannellini bean dip

makes: 4 portions

storage: up to 2–3 days in the refrigerator

1 ripe avocado, pitted and peeled
1 tsp lemon juice
400g can cannellini beans,
  drained and rinsed
2 slices bread, to serve (if your baby
  is confident with chewing)

Avocado is a great first food and is the ideal ingredient to mix with new ingredients such as cannellini beans that are slightly harder to digest. Avocados provide good mono-unsaturated fats, which will help provide your baby with energy for growing and developing, as well as useful amounts of vitamin B, which is important for a healthy nervous system.

1 Whizz the first three ingredients to a smooth purée with a hand-held blender (or in a food processor or blender).

2 Lightly toast the bread and serve in fingers spread with the purée.

vegetables in polenta

suitable from 8 months

makes: about 4 portions

storage: best eaten immediately, or up to 2–3 days in the refrigerator

1 large courgette, sliced quite thick
2 large carrots, peeled and sliced
1 free-range egg, beaten
4 tbsp polenta
2 tbsp plain flour
1 tbsp vegetarian Parmesan-style
  cheese, grated
freshly ground black pepper
3–4 tbsp vegetable oil, for frying

This is the perfect recipe for using any leftover cooked vegetables, such as grilled mushrooms, grilled aubergines, broccoli, or cauliflower. Many experts believe that some babies are ready for finger foods quite quickly after they have been weaned on to solids. This recipe is only suitable for babies who are confident with chewing.

1 Bring a pan of water to the boil and steam or boil the courgette and carrot until they are just tender. Drain and dry on absorbent kitchen paper.
2 Put the egg in a shallow bowl.
3 Mix the polenta, flour, and cheese on a large plate. Season with freshly ground black pepper.
4 Dip the vegetables into the egg, then into the polenta, and lay on a plate.
5 Heat the oil in a large frying pan and fry the vegetables briefly over a high heat until just golden and crisp. Drain on absorbent kitchen paper and serve warm as a finger food.

minestrone with herby scones

makes: 3 baby portions or 1 baby portion and 1 adult portion

storage: up to 3 days in the refrigerator

1 tbsp olive oil
2 spring onions, finely chopped
1 small carrot, peeled and finely
  diced
½ leek, finely chopped
200g tin chopped tomatoes
300ml (10½fl oz) no-salt vegetable
  stock
100g (3¼oz) tiny pasta shapes
1 tbsp freshly grated cheese, such
  as vegetarian Parmesan-style
  cheese

When using vegetable stock, make sure it is a no-salt brand because too much salt can be dangerous for small babies. If you can't find a brand without salt, just use water. Many varieties of canned tomatoes have added sugar and salt, so you should always check the labels and look for ones without these unnecessary ingredients. For the herby scones you can use the recipe for cinnamon scones (see page 105); just leave out the cinnamon and sugar, and add a large handful of finely chopped fresh herbs instead. This recipe is only suitable for babies who are confident with chewing.

1 Heat the olive oil in a large pan. Add the spring onions, carrot, and leek, and cook until the vegetables are soft and the spring onion just golden.
2 Add the tomatoes and vegetable stock and bring to the boil. Simmer for 15–20 minutes, until the vegetables are tender.
3 Add the pasta and cook until *al dente*, stirring often.
4 Stir in the grated cheese and purée until smooth.

spinach and cheese omelette

makes: 2 baby portions or 1 baby portion and 1 small adult portion

storage: best eaten immediately

3 medium free-range eggs
freshly ground black pepper
1 tbsp grated cheese, such as
  vegetarian Cheddar or Parmesan-
  style cheese
small knob of unsalted butter
50g (1¾oz) frozen petits pois or
  peas, cooked
100g (3¾oz) baby spinach leaves,
  wilted and chopped

Often parents worry about giving babies food that is too strongly flavoured, so their diets are frequently bland. Most mass-produced mild Cheddar cheese really has no discernible flavour; you don't need to go to the extremes and give them extra mature, but just choose something with a little more bite. This recipe is only suitable for babies who are confident with chewing.

1 Break the eggs into a bowl. Season with a little ground black pepper to taste and very lightly beat. Add the grated cheese.
2 Melt the butter in a heavy-based frying pan – or better still, an omelette pan – over a medium heat, then pour in the eggs. Turn up the heat and tilt the pan so that the eggs completely cover the base. Sprinkle the peas and spinach over the top of the omelette.
3 Use a wooden spoon to draw the egg mixture from the sides into the middle, then repeat, tipping the pan at the same time until the eggs are cooked. Cut into small pieces and serve.

bubble and squeak with cheese

makes: 4 baby portions or 1 baby portion and 1 large adult portions

storage: best eaten immediately

500g (1lb 2oz) potatoes, peeled and
  cut into small dice
100g (3¾oz) Savoy cabbage, finely
  shredded
50g (1¾oz) grated vegetarian
  Cheddar cheese
½ tsp wholegrain mustard
small knob of unsalted butter

A classic dish, usually made with leftovers. In fact leftovers often make perfect baby foods because cooked vegetables are quickly and easily reheated. You could make this with cabbage and any cold root vegetables, such as potatoes, parsnips, or carrots.

1 Bring a pan of water to the boil and cook the potatoes until soft (about 15 minutes).
2 Meanwhile, steam the cabbage over the top of the boiling pan for 5–6 minutes, until tender.
3 When the vegetables are done, drain them and put into a large bowl. Add the cheese and mustard. Mash with a potato masher.
4 Heat the butter in a large, heavy-based pan and add the 'bubble and squeak'. Cook over a medium heat and, using a spatula, carefully turn over when the bottom becomes golden.
5 Mash a little more or purée with a hand-held blender (or in a food processor or blender).

macaroni and cauliflower cheese

makes: 4–6 baby portions

storage: up to 2 days in the refrigerator, or up to 2 months in the freezer

100g (3¾oz) macaroni
400g (14oz) cauliflower florets
200ml (7fl oz) formula milk
20g (¾oz) plain flour
20g (¾oz) unsalted butter
freshly ground black pepper
2 tbsp finely chopped flat-leaf
  parsley
100g (3¾oz) vegetarian Cheddar,
  grated

Keep some of the tiny tender cauliflower leaves to steam with the florets and add to the dish for extra vitamins if your baby is confident with chewing.

1   Bring a pan of water to the boil and cook the macaroni until *al dente*. Cook the cauliflower over the boiling water in a steamer, until just tender (about 5 minutes). Drain and reserve.

2   Preheat the oven to 180°C/350°F/gas mark 4.

3   Mix together the milk, flour, and butter in a pan. Heat gently, stirring with a whisk, until you have a smooth sauce. Season with pepper, then add the herbs and half the cheese. Stir until the cheese has melted, then stir in the macaroni.

4   Arrange the cauliflower in an ovenproof dish. Pour over the macaroni cheese and sprinkle over the remaining cheese. Bake for 15 minutes until golden.

5   If freezing, leave to cool completely, wrap in foil, and freeze.

6   To serve, thaw thoroughly and bake at 180°C/350°F/gas mark 4 for 15–20 minutes, or until hot through, then chop into tiny pieces or mash.

creamy mushroom pasta sauce

makes: 6 baby portions

storage: 2 days in the refrigerator, or up to 2 months in the freezer

1 tbsp olive oil
3 spring onions, finely chopped
300g (10½oz) mushrooms, sliced
1 tbsp fresh parsley, finely chopped
freshly ground black pepper
100ml (3½fl oz) no-salt vegetable
  stock
50g (1¾oz) full-fat cream cheese
baby pasta or rice, cooked

Mushrooms are perennially popular with babies and young children. They shouldn't be washed because they soak up water easily – it's best to gently wipe them well with some damp absorbent kitchen paper. Try using brown cap mushrooms because they have more flavour than button mushrooms.

1   Heat the oil in a large frying pan, add the spring onions, and cook until soft and translucent (about 5 minutes).

2   Add the mushrooms and fry until they are golden and just beginning to lose their liquid. Add the parsley and black pepper, and stir well. Pour in the stock and cook over a gentle heat until the mushrooms are soft (about 4 minutes).

3   Stir in the cream cheese. If freezing, spoon into a freezer-proof container and freeze.

4   To serve, thaw thoroughly. Whizz with a hand-held blender (or in a food processor or blender) until smooth, then pour over the baby pasta or rice.

sweet potato and coconut curry

suitable from 9 months

makes: 10 baby portions

storage: up to 2 days in the refrigerator, or up to 2 months in the freezer

25g (1oz) unsalted butter
1 tbsp olive oil
1 large onion, peeled and chopped
1 garlic clove, peeled and crushed
1–2 tsp mild curry powder
1cm (½ inch) fresh ginger, peeled and finely chopped
1 small butternut squash, peeled and the flesh cut into small dice
1 small sweet potato, peeled and cut into small dice
1 large carrot, peeled and cut into small dice
200g tin chopped tomatoes
400ml (14fl oz) coconut milk
300ml (10½fl oz) no-salt vegetable stock

Older babies enjoy a creamy coconut curry. Try adding a little lime juice to give it a bit of a kick. This recipe is designed to feed the whole family, but if you only want enough for a few meals for the baby just halve the recipe. (Do not give nuts to babies if there is a family history of allergies.)

1 Heat the butter and oil in a large pan, add the onion and garlic, and cook until soft (about 5 minutes).

2 Add 1 tsp of the curry powder and the ginger, and cook for 1 minute more, stirring the mixture often. Add the butternut squash, sweet potato, and carrot, then cook for 2 minutes, stirring.

3 Add the tomatoes, coconut milk, and stock, and bring to the boil. Simmer for 15–20 minutes, until the vegetables are just tender.

4 If freezing, leave to cool completely, then spoon into a freezer-proof container. Freeze.

5 To serve, thaw thoroughly. Put into a saucepan and heat through for 10–15 minutes, or until hot through. Lightly mash or, for a smoother purée, whizz with a hand-held blender (or in a food processor or blender).

herby tomato pasta sauce

makes: 6 baby portions

storage: up to 2 days in the refrigerator, or up to 2 months in the freezer

1 tbsp olive oil
1 small onion, peeled and finely chopped
1 small garlic clove, peeled and crushed
4 fresh plum tomatoes, chopped
200g tin chopped tomatoes
2 basil leaves
freshly ground black pepper (optional)
2 tbsp fresh herbs, such as thyme, sage, parsley and rosemary, finely chopped
tiny baby pasta, cooked, to serve

This is a great freezer stand-by and can be served with noodles, rice, polenta, or even just plain old mashed potato.

1 Heat the oil in a heavy-based saucepan and fry the onion until soft and pale golden (about 5 minutes). Add the garlic and cook for 1 minute more.

2 Add the fresh and tinned tomatoes and the basil, black pepper (if using), and herbs, and simmer for 10 minutes.

3 Whizz with a hand-held blender (or in a food processor or blender) until smooth, then pass through a nylon sieve. Leave to cool, then pour into a freezer-proof container and freeze.

4 To serve, thaw thoroughly, reheat gently, and serve over cooked baby pasta.

ratatouille

makes: 6–8 baby portions

storage: up to 2 days in the refrigerator, or up to 2 months in the freezer

2 tbsp olive oil
1 medium red onion, peeled and chopped
1 small garlic clove, peeled and crushed
2 small aubergines, cut into small chunks
2 small red peppers, deseeded and chopped
2 medium courgettes
400g can chopped tomatoes
freshly ground black pepper, to taste
small sprig rosemary
tiny pasta, cooked, to serve

Another versatile dish that can be served with baked potatoes, pasta, or rice. You could also use it as the base for a vegetarian lasagne.

1 Heat the oil in a heavy-based pan and fry the onion until soft and golden (about 5 minutes). Add the garlic and aubergines and fry until soft, adding a little more oil if necessary.
2 Add the red peppers and courgettes and cook gently for 25 minutes.
3 Add the tomatoes, black pepper, and rosemary. Cover the pan with a lid and cook for another 20 minutes, stirring occasionally.
4 If freezing, leave to cool. Spoon into a freezer-proof container and freeze.
5 To serve, thaw thoroughly. Put into a saucepan and heat through for 10–15 minutes, or until hot through.
6 Remove the rosemary sprig, then chop the ratatouille finely or whizz with a hand-held blender (or in a food processor or blender) until smooth, then pour over cooked baby pasta.

sweetcorn and potato soup

makes: 10 baby portions

storage: up to 2 days in the refrigerator, or up to 2 months in the freezer

1 tbsp olive oil
10g (½oz) unsalted butter
1 small onion, peeled and finely chopped
1 small garlic clove, peeled and crushed
1 medium potato, peeled and cut into small dice
250g tin sweetcorn, drained
1 tbsp finely chopped fresh flat-leaf parsley
175ml (6fl oz) no-salt vegetable stock
125ml (4½fl oz) formula milk or calcium-enriched soy drink

If you make this soup in the summer, use a couple of new potatoes instead of a single large potato and just scrub them well instead of peeling. This will increase the fibre content of this dish, which is fine for babies who are used to solids. Also, because most of the nutrients in potatoes are stored just under the skin, they will be retained.

1 Add the oil and butter to a hot pan and fry the onion and garlic until soft and pale golden (about 5 minutes). Add the potato and cook for a further 5 minutes, stirring often. Add the sweetcorn and parsley, and stir well.
2 Pour in the stock, bring to the boil, then simmer gently for 15 minutes.
3 Whizz with a hand-held blender (or in a food processor or blender) until smooth, then pass through a nylon sieve.
4 Leave to cool. If freezing, pour in a freezer-proof container and freeze.
5 To serve, thaw thoroughly. Add the milk and reheat gently before serving.

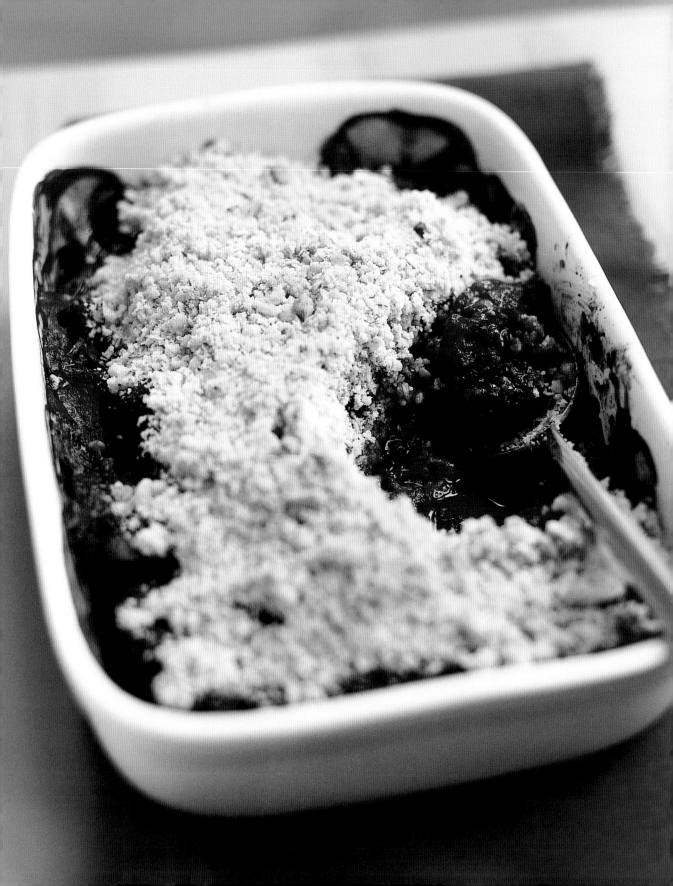

fruit dishes

7-9 months

blackberry and apple crumble

makes: 6 baby portions

storage: up to 2 days in the refrigerator, or up to 3 months in the freezer

3 medium cooking apples, such as Bramley, peeled and cored, and cut into bite-size pieces
200g (7oz) blackberries
3–4 tsp golden caster sugar (or more if the fruit is tart)
4 tbsp water

for the crumble:
100g (3¾oz) plain flour
50g (1¾oz) unsalted butter
50g (1¾oz) porridge oats
2 tsp golden caster sugar
pinch of ground cinnamon

This recipe is not suitable for babies who are not confident with chewing.

1 Put the apples into a pan with the blackberries, sugar, and water. Heat gently until the berries are just starting to give up their juice.

2 For the crumble, put the flour into a bowl and rub in the butter until the mixture resembles breadcrumbs. Stir in the oats, sugar, and cinnamon.

3 Put the fruit in a shallow ovenproof dish or into five or six small ramekins. If freezing, leave to cool, then cover and freeze. Put the crumble mix in a freezer bag and freeze.

4 To serve, thaw the fruit and crumble mixture thoroughly. You will need 4–5 tbsp crumble mix for each small ramekin. Preheat the oven to 180°C/350°F/gas mark 4. Sprinkle the crumble over the fruit and bake in the oven for 25 minutes, until the crumble is crisp and golden on top. Lightly mash if necessary.

orchard fruit with ground nuts

makes: 5–6 portions

storage: up to 2–3 days in the refrigerator

3 apples, peeled, cored, and thinly sliced
200g (7oz) blackberries (or raspberries, blackcurrants, or blueberries)
20g (¾oz) ground almonds

If you are making this in the autumn, use blackberries with the apple. During summer, make the most of summer berries such as raspberries or blueberries. You can serve this swirled into custard or yogurt, or mixed with cereal to make it slightly more filling. (Do not feed nuts to babies if there is any family history of allergies.)

1 Put the apple and all the berries into a saucepan with 1 tbsp water.

2 Cook over a gentle heat for 2–3 minutes until the fruit starts to release juice and the apple is soft. Remove from the heat and leave to cool.

3 Stir in the ground almonds. Purée or lightly mash if necessary.

vanilla rice pudding

makes: 2–3 baby portions plus
1–2 adult portions

storage: best eaten immediately, or up
to 1–2 days in the refrigerator. (Rice
should not be reheated, but can be
served cold.)

150g (5½oz) short-grain
  (pudding) rice
500ml full-fat milk or soy milk
100ml (3½fl oz) water
½ vanilla pod, split lengthways or
  ½ tsp vanilla extract
1–2 tbsp golden caster sugar (or
  preferably omit)
1 small knob of unsalted butter
½ ripe medium banana, roughly
  chopped (or handful of berries)

If possible, try to buy the organic version of some of the foods on your
shopping list. Organic cows' milk is one of the most widely available organic
foods and one with the most markedly difference in flavour to its non-
organic equivalent – sweet and clean without the chemical overtones of
ordinary milk. This is because organic herds are fed only natural foodstuffs;
the use of animal-derived feed is prohibited.

1 Put the rice, milk, water, and vanilla into a saucepan and stir.
2 Bring to the boil, then reduce the heat and simmer for 15–20 minutes,
   stirring often to prevent the mixture from sticking. If necessary, add a few
   more tablespoons of water to the mixture.
3 Add the sugar, if using, and butter. Mix well and cook for another minute.
   Remove the vanilla pod if using. Mash if necessary. This is good warm or cold
   served with chopped banana or small berries.

dried fruit purée with yogurt

suitable from 9 months

makes: 4–5 portions or 2–3 baby
portions and 1–2 adult portions

storage: up to 2–3 days in the
refrigerator

100ml (3½fl oz) apple juice
50g (1¾oz) dried apricots, pitted
  and finely chopped
50g (1¾oz) ready-to-eat dates,
  pitted and finely chopped
1 ripe banana, sliced
200ml (7fl oz) natural full-fat
  yogurt

Use any dried fruits that you have to hand; look out for medjool dates – they
are really plump and delicious. Dates are a great source of fibre and help to
prevent your baby from getting constipated. They are also rich in potassium,
which helps to maintain your baby's fluid balance. You make also like to mix
this purée with a little breakfast cereal for your baby, and you may enjoy a
dollop on top of your own breakfast cereal at the same time!

1 Put the apple juice in a small pan. Add the dried fruits, checking for any
   stones that may be left.
2 Bring to the boil, take off the heat and leave for at least 30 minutes.
3 Whizz with the other ingredients using a hand-held blender (or in a food
   processor or blender) until the purée is smooth.

stewed rhubarb scones

makes: about 10

storage: keep the scones in an airtight container for up to 1 week or up to 3 months in the freezer. Keep the stewed rhubarb for up to 2–3 days in the refrigerator or up to 3 months in the freezer

a little unsalted butter

for the cinnamon scones:
200g (7oz) self-raising flour
½ tsp baking powder
½ tsp ground cinnamon
1 tbsp golden caster sugar
4 tbsp sour cream
1 free-range egg
75ml (2½fl oz) full-fat milk

for the stewed rhubarb:
4 large sticks rhubarb, chopped
50ml (2fl oz) apple juice
200g (7oz) raspberries

These scones are ideal for babies as they are not too sweet. They make a great pudding or are ideal for breakfast served with fresh fruit. A little apple juice and some raspberries should be enough to sweeten the rhubarb without the need for any sugar. Remember babies find foods much sweeter than we do. Only serve scones to babies who are confident with chewing.

1 Preheat the oven to 200°C/400°F/gas mark 6. Lightly butter a baking sheet.
2 Sieve the flour, baking powder, and cinnamon into a bowl. Stir in the sugar, then make a well in the middle.
3 In a separate bowl, mix together the sour cream, egg, and milk, and pour into the dry ingredients. Mix together, but do not beat.
4 Drop 10 tsp of the mixture onto a the baking sheet and bake for 12–14 minutes, until risen and golden. Cool on a wire rack.
5 Wash the rhubarb and cut into 2.5cm (1 inch) pieces. Put into a buttered ovenproof dish. Sprinkle over the apple juice and bake for 15 minutes. Add the raspberries, cover with foil, and bake for a further 10 minutes or until the rhubarb is tender, but still in pieces. Leave to cool completely. Pour into freezer-proof containers and freeze. Thaw completely before heating through in a saucepan. Serve the scones with the stewed fruit.

strawberry and apple purée

makes: 3 baby portions, or 1 baby portion and 1 adult portion as a smoothie base or cereal topping

storage: best eaten immediately

½ small eating apple, such as Cox's orange pippin, peeled, cored, and roughly chopped
handful of strawberries, hulled
1 mint leaf

Mint goes really well with strawberries, but try adding it to other fruit purées, too, especially melon. This is a great purée to give a baby who may be constipated, because strawberries are rich in both soluble and insoluble fibre, which help to relieve the condition.

1 Put the apple into a small saucepan with 2 tbsp water and heat gently until the apple is soft and pulpy.
2 Cool, then add the strawberries and mint. Whizz with a hand-held blender (or in a food processor or blender) until smooth.

plum yogurt with muesli

makes: 2 baby portions

storage: best eaten immediately or up to 24 hours in the refrigerator

1 ripe plum, such as Victoria or greengage, pitted and roughly chopped
tiny pinch of ground ginger
2 tbsp natural full-fat yogurt
1 tbsp ground baby muesli
breast milk or formula milk, to serve

Small amounts of spices can be added to lots of different purées not only to make them more interesting to your baby, but also to educate her palate. It is at this early stage that a lifetime's eating habits can be influenced, so be bold! You could also include a little fresh grated ginger instead of ground ginger. Avoid muesli that contains nuts if there is any family history of allergies.

1 Put the plum in a saucepan with the ginger and 2 tbsp water, and heat gently until the plum is soft. Leave to cool.

2 Mash the plum into a purée, then add the yogurt, muesli, and enough breast milk or formula milk to create the desired consistency. Mix together well and mash if necessary.

prune and banana porridge

suitable from 9 months

makes: 3 baby portions, or 1 baby portion and 1 adult portion

storage: best eaten immediately, or up to 24 hours in the refrigerator

125ml (4½fl oz) boiling water
2 prunes, pitted and finely chopped
200ml (7fl oz) breast milk or formula milk
60g (2oz) oats
½ ripe medium banana, roughly chopped

A great purée for any older baby who is prone to constipation because prunes are a natural laxative. But dried fruits can be difficult to digest, so I'd advise keeping this one for babies who are 9 months or older. As with all fruit for babies, make sure the bananas are ripe – they should have black spots. Unripe bananas can be indigestible for babies, as well as causing wind.

1 Pour the boiling water over the prunes, then leave them to soak for 30 minutes.

2 Put the soaked prunes in a pan with all the other ingredients except the banana, then heat on a low heat for 5 minutes, stirring often, until the mixture has thickened.

3 Add the banana and purée with a hand-blender (or in a food processor), adding a little more milk or cooled, boiled water to thin, if necessary.

apple and banana purée

makes: 2 baby portions

storage: best eaten immediately, or up to 24 hours in the refrigerator

1 small eating apple, such as Cox's orange pippin, peeled, cored, and chopped into small pieces
1 small ripe banana, roughly chopped

This simple purée is always a favourite with babies, who love the taste of banana and the sweetness of apple.

1 Put the apple in a pan with a little boiling water (about 75ml/2½fl oz) and simmer gently until the apple is soft and pulpy (about 5 minutes), adding a little more water if necessary. Cool.
2 Whizz the banana and apple mixture together using a hand-held blender (or in a food processor or blender) until smooth.

raspberry and blueberry compote

makes: 3–4 baby portions

storage: up to 2–3 days in the refrigerator, or up to 2 months in the freezer

200g (7oz) raspberries, fresh or frozen
200g (7oz) fresh blueberries
6 tbsp water

Always pick over soft fruit for leaves and bugs – the easiest way to do this is to lay them on something white, such as absorbent kitchen paper. In the autumn, look out for bilberries, a type of blueberry that has a distinctive bright-blue juice and a delicious flavour.

1 Put the raspberries and blueberries into a small saucepan with the water. Heat gently until just simmering and cook until all the fruit has burst and the raspberries are pulpy.
2 Remove from the heat and cool before whizzing with a hand-held blender (or in a food processor or blender).
3 Spoon the purée into ice-cube trays. If freezing, cover with foil or put into a freezer bag and seal. Freeze.
4 To serve, thaw thoroughly.

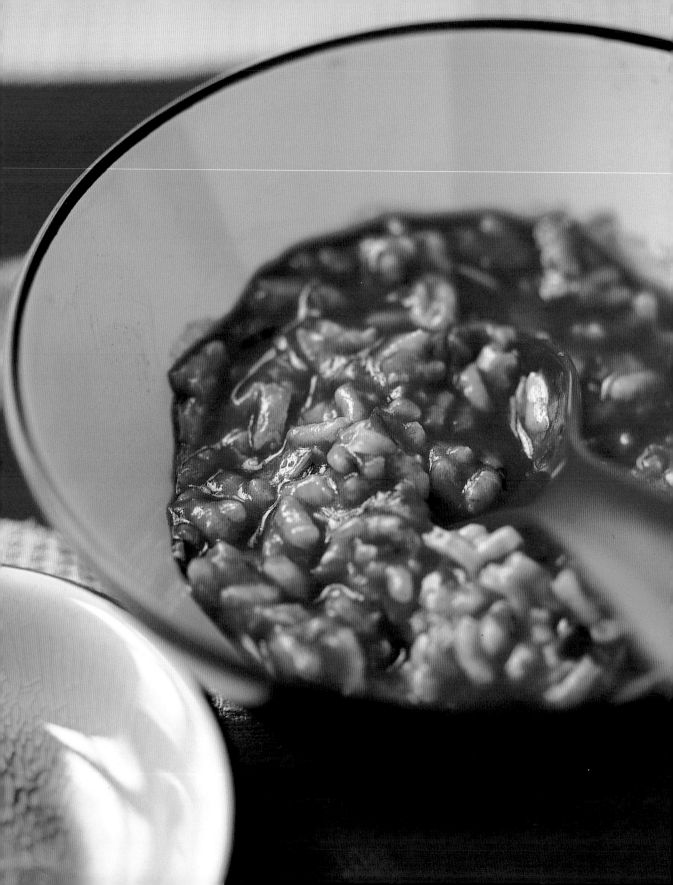

vegetarian savouries
10-12 months

tomato risotto

makes: 6 baby portions, or 2 baby portions and 2 adult portions

storage: best eaten immediately, or up to 1-2 days in the refrigerator. (Rice should not be reheated, but can be served cold)

25g (1oz) unsalted butter
3 shallots, finely chopped
175g (6oz) arborio rice
300ml (10½fl oz) tomato passata or tinned chopped tomatoes
475ml (17fl oz) light no-salt vegetable stock (very weak)
2 tbsp fresh basil, torn into small pieces
50g (1¾oz) vegetarian Parmesan-style cheese, grated

This risotto is particularly easy because constant stirring isn't required – you just bung it in the oven.

1 Preheat the oven at 180°C/350°F/gas mark 4.
2 Melt the butter in a heavy-based pan and fry the shallots slowly, without colouring, until softened (about 5–10 minutes). Turn the heat up slightly, then add the rice to the pan and stir, coating it with the shallots.
3 Stir for 1–2 minutes, until you hear the rice make a hissing sound, which means it's time to add the liquid. Add the tomato passata and stir. Let it bubble, then add the stock and 1 tbsp of the basil. Bring up to simmering point, stir once, and transfer to an uncovered warm ovenproof dish. Put in the middle of the oven. After 20 minutes, remove and stir once.
4 Return to the oven for 15 minutes. When the rice is cooked but has a little bite, stir in the cheese and remaining basil. Leave for 2 minutes, cool, then serve.

scrambled eggs and toasted bun

makes: 1 baby portion

storage: best eaten immediately

small knob of unsalted butter
2 large free-range eggs
2–3 tbsp full-fat milk or calcium-enriched soy drink
freshly ground black pepper (optional)
1 tbsp chopped fresh herbs (optional)
1 wholemeal bun
unsalted butter, for spreading

Scrambled eggs is one of the quickest and most versatile meals for the entire family – this could just as easily be served for lunch, supper or breakfast. Keeping it simple is often best, but you can add lots of things to scrambled eggs: peas, chopped herbs (especially chives), mushrooms – the list is endless.

1 Melt the butter in a non-stick pan. Whisk the eggs and milk together, and season with a little black pepper and fresh herbs, if using.
2 Pour the eggs into the pan and cook over a gentle heat, stirring constantly until they are scrambled and well cooked, with no runny bits.
3 Slice the bun in half and toast until just pale golden, then spread with a little butter.
4 Cut one half of the bun into small pieces. Top with half the scrambled egg. Serve the remaining bun and scrambled egg on a plate for you.

eastern rice with baby veg

makes: 4 baby portions, or 2 baby portions and 2 adult portions

storage: best eaten immediately, or up to 1–2 days in the refrigerator. (Rice should not be reheated.)

3 mange-tout
3 baby carrots
3 baby corn
200g (7oz) basmati rice
400ml (14fl oz) water
10g (½oz) creamed coconut
4 cardamom pods
1 cinnamon stick
squeeze of lime juice
handful of chopped fresh coriander (optional)

Do not serve coconut to babies if there is any family history of allergies.

1   Thinly slice the mange-tout, baby carrots, and baby corn into even-size pieces to make sure that they cook evenly.
2   Put the rice, water, creamed coconut, cardamom pods, and cinnamon stick into a saucepan, stir well, then cover and bring up to simmering point. Simmer for 11 minutes without removing the lid.
3   Remove the pan from the heat. Throw the sliced vegetables on top of the rice and quickly replace the lid, then cook for another 14 minutes.
4   Remove the cardamom pods and cinnamon stick. Add the lime juice, toss everything together and scatter in a little fresh coriander, if using. Mash if necessary.

leek and broccoli crumble

makes: 2–3 baby portions and 2 adult portions

storage: up to 2–3 days in the refrigerator or up to 3 months in the freezer

a little unsalted butter
3 leeks, cut into bite-size pieces
3 carrots, peeled and cut into bite-size pieces
1 head of broccoli, cut into small florets
50g (1¾oz) unsalted butter
50g (1¾oz) plain flour
600ml (21fl oz) full-fat milk
freshly ground black pepper
150g (5½oz) vegetarian Cheddar, grated
50g (1¾oz) hazelnuts or walnuts, finely chopped
30g (1oz) sunflower seeds
50g (1¾oz) wholemeal breadcrumbs
2 tbsp fresh flat-leaf parsley, finely chopped

Introduce the darker green vegetables such as broccoli as early as possible and your baby will be less likely to develop an aversion to them later. Broccoli is an excellent source of vitamin C and it also contains betacarotene, which your baby's body will convert into vitamin A, together with folate, iron, and potassium. (Do not feed nuts to babies if there is any family history of allergies.)

1   Butter an ovenproof dish. Steam or boil the vegetables until just tender – they should still have a bit of bite. Drain well and put into an ovenproof dish.
2   Preheat the oven to 180°C/350°F/gas mark 4. Melt the butter in a saucepan, add the flour, and stir over a medium heat for 1 minute. Remove from the heat and add the milk gradually, stirring constantly until smooth.
3   Return the pan to the heat and slowly bring to the boil, stirring constantly, until the sauce is smooth and thick. Season with black pepper, remove from the heat, and stir in nearly all the cheese, reserving 2 tbsp for the topping.
4   To make the crumble, mix together the remaining cheese, nuts, seeds, breadcrumbs, and parsley. Season with black pepper.
5   Pour the cheese sauce over the vegetables. Sprinkle over the crumble topping. If freezing, leave to cool completely. Pour into freezer-proof containers and freeze. Thaw completely before heating in a saucepan.
6   Cook for 25 minutes until the top is golden and the sauce is bubbling. Finely chop or mash.

cheese and corn muffins

makes: 15 baby portions

storage: up to 2–3 days in the refrigerator, or up to 3 months in the freezer

100g (3¾oz) tin sweetcorn
150g (5½oz) plain flour
½ tsp baking powder
1 large free-range egg
125ml (4½fl oz) full-fat milk
50g (1¾oz) unsalted butter, melted
50g (1¾oz) vegetarian Cheddar, grated
pinch of mild chilli powder
1 tbsp chopped fresh flat-leaf parsley

These muffins are popular with children of all ages. Serve them with cheese and chopped tomato and avocado. They are also good served with soup.

1 Preheat the oven to 200°C/400°F/gas mark 6. Grease a mini-muffin tin or line with paper cases. Drain and mash the sweetcorn.

2 Sift the flour and baking powder into a bowl. In another bowl, mix together the egg, milk, melted butter, cheese, sweetcorn, chilli, and parsley.

3 Pour the flour mixture over the wet ingredients and quickly fold in. Don't overmix: it should look lumpy. Spoon into the tin and bake for 15 minutes until risen and golden. If freezing, cool on a wire rack and freeze in a freezer-proof container.

4 To serve, heat through from frozen in a pre-heated oven at 180°C/350°F/gas mark 4 for 5–6 minutes. Break into very small pieces.

bean and herb sausages

makes: 14 sausages

storage: 2–3 days in the refrigerator or up to 3 months in the freezer

420g can haricot or cannellini beans and 1 tbsp tomato paste, or 400g tin baked beans
100g (3¾oz) soft brown breadcrumbs
45g (1½oz) vegetarian Cheddar, grated
1 free-range egg, lightly beaten
1 small onion, finely chopped
1 tbsp chopped fresh herbs of your choice, such as thyme, parsley
1 tbsp lemon juice
dried breadcrumbs
vegetable oil, for frying

for the tomato relish:
200g (7oz) ripe tomatoes, finely chopped
¼ red onion, peeled and very finely chopped
½ clove garlic, peeled and crushed
¼ red pepper, very finely chopped
2 tbsp olive oil
2 tsp red wine vinegar

If you are using baked beans in this recipe, try to choose organic beans that do not have any added salt. These 'sausages' are an ideal finger food that your baby can grab hold of and dip into the relish.

1 Put the beans in a bowl and mash with a fork. Add the breadcrumbs, cheese, egg, onion, herbs, and lemon juice and mix together thoroughly. Season with freshly ground black pepper. Form the mixture into 18–20 sausages about 10cm (4 inches) long.

2 Roll the sausages in dried breadcrumbs and chill in the refrigerator for 30 minutes. If freezing, leave to cool completely. Pour into freezer-proof containers and freeze. Thaw thoroughly.

3 Meanwhile make the relish. Mix all the ingredients together in a bowl and refrigerate.

4 Heat a frying pan with a little oil and cook the sausages for 2–3 minutes before turning, then cook for another 6–8 minutes, turning frequently to ensure that they brown evenly. Drain on absorbent kitchen paper and serve, if necessary chopped into small pieces, with the tomato relish.

peanut butter eggy bread

makes: 4 portions

storage: best eaten immediately

about 4 tbsp peanut butter
4 slices wholemeal bread
1 free-range egg
100ml (3½fl oz) full-fat milk
20g (¾oz) butter
1 tbsp olive oil

Eggs are not only a good source of protein, but also the yolks are high in minerals – among them zinc, calcium, and iron. They also contain vitamins A, D and B. If possible, try to choose good-quality wholemeal bread from a baker, rather than factory-made bread, and use organic peanut butter, or at least a brand that has very little – preferably no – added salt or sugar. (Do not feed nuts to babies if there is any family history of allergies.)

1 Spread the peanut butter on one side of each of the slices of bread.
2 Mix the egg and milk together in a shallow dish and dip the bread into this eggy mixture.
3 Heat the oil and butter in a frying pan and fry the dipped bread, turning over after 2–3 minutes, so each side is golden brown. Cut into small pieces if necessary.

Moroccan chickpea stew

makes: 2 baby portions and 2 adult portions

storage: 2–3 days in the refrigerator

for the couscous:
200g (7oz) couscous
250ml (9fl oz) boiling water

4 tbsp olive oil
1 large Spanish onion, peeled and
  grated or very finely chopped
1 large potato, peeled and diced
1 clove garlic, peeled and crushed
¼ tsp ground ginger
¼ tsp ground cinnamon
¼ tsp ground cumin (optional)
6 dried apricots, very finely chopped
400g tin plum tomatoes
400g tin chickpeas, rinsed
500ml (18fl oz) no-salt vegetable
  stock
freshly ground black pepper
handful of fresh coriander or
  parsley, chopped

Introduce chickpeas gradually or they can be overwhelming for a baby's immature digestive system. Pulses are notorious for their 'windiness', but as long as they are well cooked you should have no problems. Interestingly, some believe that a little parsley can help to counteract this side effect, so you may choose to add a little of this herb, rather than coriander.

1 Put the couscous into a heatproof bowl. Pour over the boiling water and cover with a plate. Leave for at least 15 minutes.
2 Heat the oil in a large heavy-based pan. Add the onion and fry over a medium heat until soft and just starting to colour. Add the potato and fry until golden brown.
3 Turn the heat up a little and add the garlic, ginger, cinnamon, cumin (if using), and apricots, and cook for 2–3 minutes, stirring constantly.
4 Add the tomatoes, chickpeas and vegetable stock. Bring to the boil, cover, and simmer gently for 15 minutes, until the potatoes are cooked.
5 Season with black pepper and add the fresh coriander. Mash if necessary. Fluff up the couscous with a fork and serve with the Moroccan stew.

hot carrot salad

makes: 4 portions

storage: best eaten immediately, or keep the carrot salad and cottage cheese separately for up to 2–3 days in the refrigerator

50g (1¾oz) raisins
juice of 1 orange
small knob of unsalted butter
6 large carrots, coarsely grated
freshly ground black pepper
100g (3¾oz) sunflower seeds,
  toasted
200g (7oz) full-fat vegetarian
  cottage cheese
4 slices granary toast

If you think that your baby may prefer the texture of raw carrots, then simply mix the grated carrots with the soaked raisins, instead of cooking the carrot first, and perhaps use a little less fresh orange juice. (Do not feed nuts to babies if there is any family history of allergies.)

1   Soak the raisins in the orange juice for at least 30 minutes.
2   Meanwhile, heat the butter in a frying pan over a low heat and cook the carrots, stirring gently: it will take about 3–4 minutes. Add the raisins and orange juice, and turn the heat up and cook until the orange juice has evaporated.
3   Remove from the heat and season with a little black pepper.
4   Sprinkle the toasted seeds over the cottage cheese. Serve the hot salad with the cottage cheese and toast. You may find it easier to spread the cottage cheese on the toast and top with some of the carrot.

egg-fried rice with peas

makes: 4 portions

storage: best eaten immediately, or up to 1–2 days in the refrigerator. (Rice should not be reheated, but can be served cold)

1 cup basmati rice
2 tbsp vegetable oil
1 clove garlic, peeled and crushed
2 large carrots, peeled and coarsely
  grated
100g (3¾oz) mange-tout, sliced
  diagonally
150g (5½oz) frozen peas
2 free-range eggs, beaten
few dashes of soy sauce (optional)

This dish has a great texture for babies with its contrast of soft egg rice and slightly crunchy vegetables. Rice, like most cereals, is a good source of energy, containing large amounts of starch. It is a staple food in many parts of the world, supplying protein, fibre, vitamins, and minerals. Add any vegetables that you have to hand and chop them to the size most suitable for your baby.

1   Put 1 cup of rice into a pan and add 2 cups of water. (The exact size for the cup does not matter as long as you use the same cup for measuring the rice and the water.) Cover and bring to the boil, lower the heat, and simmer gently for exactly 14 minutes. Take off the heat and leave, still covered, for a further 11 minutes.
2   Heat the oil in a wok or large frying pan. Add the garlic and sauté gently until just soft.
3   Add the carrots and mange-tout, and cook for 2 minutes, stirring often. Add the peas and rice, and cook for 1 minute more, stirring often.
4   Add the eggs and cook over a high heat, stirring constantly until the egg is cooked and golden in places.
5   Chop into small pieces. Serve immediately.

sweet potato hummus

makes: 3 baby portions

storage: 48 hours in the refrigerator

2 medium sweet potatoes, well
   scrubbed
400g tin chickpeas, drained
   and rinsed
1 tbsp tahini
1 garlic clove, peeled and chopped
juice of ½ lemon
1 tbsp olive oil

to serve:
a few fingers of pitta bread
   (optional)
selection of soft vegetables for
   dipping, such as peeled cucumber
   or cooked beetroot, cut into sticks

This is fantastic for mums and dads, as well as babies. Chickpeas are one of the most nutritionally valuable pulses, and a great source of protein for vegetarians, so canned chickpeas are a useful store-cupboard ingredient. (Do not serve tahini to babies if there is any family history of allergies.)

1 Preheat oven to 190°C/375°F/gas mark 5.
2 Score a cross in each sweet potato and bake until they are soft and tender (about 40 minutes).
3 Scoop the potato flesh into a food processor, discarding the skins. Add the chickpeas, tahini, and garlic, and whizz together. Add the lemon juice and enough oil to make the desired consistency.
4 Serve with toasted fingers of pitta bread, if using, and soft vegetable sticks.

veggie burgers

makes: 8 baby portions

storage: up to 2–3 days in the refrigerator, or up to 2 months in the freezer

450g (1lb) potatoes, peeled and cut
   into chunks
30g (1oz) unsalted butter
200g (7oz) cooked vegetables, such
   as carrots, courgettes, peas,
   leeks – all well drained
50g (1¾oz) tinned butter beans,
   drained, rinsed, and mashed
2 tbsp finely chopped fresh herbs,
   such as parsley, thyme
50g (1¾oz) vegetarian Cheddar,
   grated
freshly ground black pepper
1 large free-range egg, beaten
90g (3½oz) dried breadcrumbs
vegetable oil, for frying

Store-bought veggie burgers are often one of the most disappointing convenience foods. These are easy to make and freeze really well, so it's worth making a double batch.

1 Cook the potatoes in boiling water until tender (about 10 minutes). Drain and mash with the butter.
2 Stir in the cooked vegetables, mashed butter beans, herbs, cheese, and pepper.
3 Using your hands (wet hands are probably easiest), form the mixture into approximately 16 balls, then flatten into patties.
4 Dip each patty in beaten egg, then into breadcrumbs, making sure each side is well covered, then lay on a plate. If freezing, layer with greaseproof paper in a freezerproof container. Freeze. Thaw thoroughly on absorbent kitchen paper.
5 Pour enough oil into a frying pan just to cover the bottom. Fry the patties over a medium heat until golden on both sides (about 6–8 minutes). Blot on kitchen paper and serve immediately. If necessary, finely chop or mash before serving.

squash gratin

makes: 4 baby portions

storage: up to 2–3 days in the refrigerator, or up to 2 months in freezer

1 small leek, finely sliced
25g (1oz) unsalted butter
1 small onion, peeled and chopped
1 garlic clove, peeled and crushed
500g (1lb 2oz) butternut squash flesh, peeled and in small cubes
200ml (7fl oz) tomato passata
200ml (7fl oz) water or no-salt vegetable stock
4 tbsp natural Greek yogurt
freshly ground black pepper
knob of unsalted butter
100g (3¾oz) breadcrumbs
100g (3¾oz) vegetarian Cheddar, grated

This is a yummy winter dish. Adults will enjoy this as a lunch on its own or as an accompaniment to something more substantial. If you have any sage growing in your garden, a little would be a great addition to this dish.

1 Wash the leek. Heat the butter in a heavy-based frying pan and fry the onion, leek, and garlic until soft (about 5 minutes). Add the squash and cook over a low heat for another 5 minutes, stirring often.

2 Add the tomato passata and water, then simmer for 10–15 minutes, until the squash is just soft. Stir in the yogurt and black pepper.

3 Pour into a buttered ovenproof dish. Melt the knob of butter in a pan, add the breadcrumbs, and stir well. Sprinkle the buttery breadcrumbs and grated cheese over the top of the squash mixture.

4 If freezing, leave to cool, then wrap with foil or cling film and freeze. Thaw thoroughly. Bake at 180°C/350°F/gas mark 4 for 40 minutes, until the top is crisp and golden. Finely chop or mash before serving.

mini quiches

makes: 6 baby portions

storage: up to 2–3 days in the refrigerator, or up to 2 months in the freezer

for the pastry:
175g (6oz) plain flour, sieved
90g (3½oz) unsalted butter, cut into small pieces and kept in the refrigerator
1 free-range egg yolk plus 1 tbsp cold water, or 2–4 tbsp cold water

for the fillings:
15g (½oz) unsalted butter
1 small onion, peeled and finely chopped
125g (4½oz) courgettes, thinly sliced
125g (4½oz) broccoli, in small pieces
50g (1¾oz) vegetarian Gruyère, grated
2 large free-range eggs plus 1 extra free-range egg yolk
270ml (9½fl oz) full-fat milk

These can be made with different fillings – use whatever you have to hand.

1 Put the flour into a food processor and whizz for a minute to aerate. Add the butter and whizz until the mixture resembles fine breadcrumbs.

2 Add the egg yolk and cold water, if necessary, and whizz until the pastry draws together. Turn on to a floured surface and knead to form a flat round.

3 Use the pastry to line six chilled 10cm (4 inch) quiche tins, trim the edges, and chill for 1 hour. Preheat the oven to 190°C/375°F/gas mark 5. Cover the pastry cases with baking parchment and baking beans, and bake blind for 5 minutes. Remove the paper and beans, and cook until just light golden (about 5 minutes). Remove from the oven and reduce the heat.

4 For the filling, heat the butter in a frying pan and soften the onion for 5 minutes. Add the courgettes and brown a little, turning frequently. Spoon into the pastry cases with the broccoli and top with the grated cheese.

5 Beat the eggs and yolk, then whisk in the milk. Pour over the filling, place the quiches on a baking sheet, and bake until the centres are set and the fillings are golden and puffy (20–25 minutes). Cool slightly, then serve.

6 If freezing, leave to cool, wrap in foil, and freeze. Thaw thoroughly, then bake at 180°C/350°F/gas mark 4 for 5 minutes. If necessary, finely chop or mash before serving.

roasted vegetable lasagne

makes: 2–3 baby portions and 4 adult portions

storage: up to 2–3 days in the refrigerator or up to 3 months in the freezer

for the sauce:
55g (2oz) unsalted butter
40g (1½oz) plain flour
580ml (20½fl oz) full-fat milk
150g (5½oz) vegetarian Cheddar, grated

2 medium aubergines, finely diced
2 courgettes, finely chopped
2 red onions, peeled and finely chopped
1 red pepper, halved, seeded and finely chopped
200g (7oz) cherry tomatoes, halved
2 cloves garlic, peeled and crushed
2 tbsp olive oil
400g tin chopped tomatoes
freshly ground black pepper, to taste
few fresh basil leaves, torn
10–12 lasagne sheets
3 tbsp freshly grated vegetarian Parmesan-style cheese

There are so many ways of making vegetarian lasagne, but I find this is an ideal way to feed babies a wide variety of vegetables.

1 Preheat the oven to 200°C/400°F/gas mark 6. Butter a large ovenproof dish or four small ovenproof dishes.

2 Put the aubergines, courgettes, onions, peppers, cherry tomatoes, and garlic into a roasting tin. Drizzle over the oil and roast for 30 minutes, turning once. Take the roasting tin out of the oven and add the tin of tomatoes, season with a little black pepper, and scatter over the torn basil leaves.

3 Lower the oven temperature to 180°C/350°F/gas mark 4. For the sauce, melt the butter in a saucepan and add the flour. Cook for 1 minute. Remove the pan from the heat and gradually add the milk, stirring constantly. Return to the heat and slowly bring to the boil, stirring constantly, until the sauce is smooth and thick. Season, remove from the heat and stir in the Cheddar.

4 Spoon some of the roasted vegetable mixture into the bottom of the ovenproof dish, then cover with a single layer of lasagne sheets. Spoon a third of the cheese sauce over the lasagne. Repeat this process, ending with a layer of cheese sauce. Sprinkle the cheese over the top. If freezing, leave to cool completely. Pour into freezer-proof containers and freeze. Thaw completely before heating through.

5 Bake in the oven for 25–30 minutes until golden and the pasta is cooked. Chop into small pieces.

curried parsnip and pear soup

makes: 10 baby portions

storage: up to 2–3 days in the refrigerator, or up to 3 months in the freezer

1 tbsp olive oil
25g (1oz) unsalted butter
1 small onion, peeled and chopped
1 garlic clove, peeled and chopped
1 medium potato, peeled, chopped
600g (1lb 6oz) parsnips, peeled and chopped
1 tsp mild curry powder
1 litre (1¾ pints) water
1 ripe pear, peeled, cored, and chopped
300ml (10½fl oz) full-fat milk

Try serving this with some warm, Indian-style bread, such as naan, which is soft and easy for babies to chew. This is quite a thick soup, which should make it slightly easier for your baby to eat without making too much of a mess.

1 Heat the oil and butter in a heavy-based saucepan.

2 Fry the onion and garlic until soft, then add the potato, parsnips, and curry powder, and cook for a further 1–2 minutes. Stir the mixture to prevent it sticking to the pan.

3 Add the water and pear and bring up to the boil. Simmer gently for 20 minutes, until the parsnip is soft.

4 Blend with a hand-held blender (or in a food processor or blender) until really smooth. If freezing, freeze in a freezer-proof container or freezer bags.

5 To serve, thaw thoroughly, add the milk, and reheat gently in a saucepan without boiling.

mild lentil curry

makes: 8 portions

storage: up to 2–3 days in the refrigerator or up to 3 months in the freezer

2 tbsp vegetable oil
1 large onion, peeled and chopped
1.5cm (½ inch) piece fresh ginger, peeled and very finely chopped
2 cloves garlic, peeled and crushed
1 tbsp mild Madras curry powder
1 small cauliflower, cut into florets
3 large carrots, peeled and cut into bite-sized pieces
1 red pepper, deseeded and sliced
1 large potato, peeled and roughly chopped
225g (8oz) tomatoes, finely chopped
100g (3¾oz) split red lentils
250ml (9fl oz) no-salt vegetable stock
400ml (14fl oz) coconut milk
4 tbsp natural Greek yogurt
large handful of fresh coriander leaves, chopped
rice, to serve

I gave mild curries to all three of my children when they were this age, and they have all enjoyed a little 'spice' since. Recipes such as this are great way of enticing babies to eat lots of vegetables in one sitting! (Do not feed nuts to babies if there is any family history of allergies.)

1 Heat the oil in a large frying pan and fry the onion until soft and pale golden. Add the garlic and ginger, and cook for 1 minute, stirring often. Add the curry powder and cook for 2–3 minutes, stirring constantly.

2 Add the cauliflower, carrots, pepper, and potato, and stir well so all the pieces are coated. Stir in the tomatoes, lentils, stock, and coconut milk.

3 Stir gently, bring to the boil, cover, and simmer gently for 25–30 minutes until the vegetables are tender.

4 Remove from the heat and stir in the yogurt and coriander. Purée with a hand-held blender (or in a food processor or blender) if you need to, or chop into smaller pieces. Serve with rice. If freezing, leave to cool completely. Pour into freezer-proof containers and freeze. Thaw completely before heating through. Do not reheat rice.

Spanish tortilla

makes: 4 baby portions, or 2 baby portions and 1 adult portion

storage: best eaten immediately or up to 24 hours in the refrigerator

450g (1lb) floury potatoes, peeled and halved
2 tbsp olive oil
1 onion, peeled and thinly sliced
4 large free-range eggs, beaten

This delicious potato omelette is wonderful with some quickly sautéed mushrooms to help to make it a little more substantial.

1 Bring a pan of water to the boil.

2 Boil the potatoes until they are soft on the outside, but still firm in the middle (about 5–7 minutes). Drain and cut into thin slices.

3 Heat the olive oil in a frying pan and add the onion. Cook slowly for 10 minutes until the onion is soft. Add the potato and cook for a further 5 minutes.

4 Preheat the grill to high.

5 Pour the beaten eggs over the potato and onion mixture and cook over a medium heat until it has set on the bottom. Put the pan under the grill to finish cooking the top.

6 Cut a quarter of the omelette into small pieces.

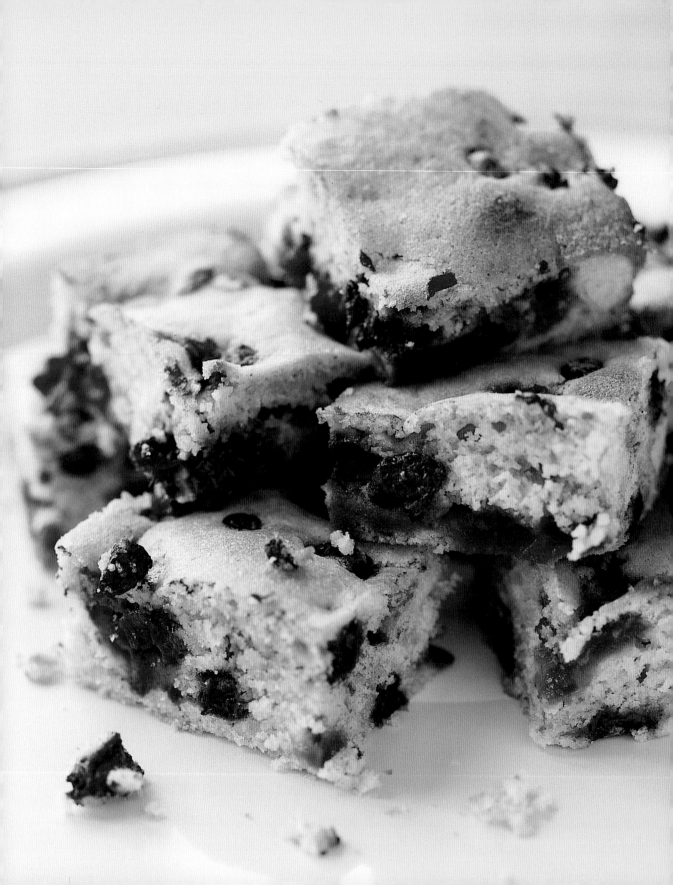

fruit dishes

10-12 months

berry sponge

makes: 10 baby portions

storage: in an airtight container for 3-4 days, or up to 3 months in the freezer

125g (4½oz) unsalted butter, softened
75g (2½oz) golden caster sugar
2 free-range eggs, lightly beaten
2 drops vanilla extract
125g (4½oz) self-raising flour
175g (6oz) mixed berries, such as blueberries, raspberries, cherries (pitted), fresh or frozen

If you can't get hold of any fresh berries, use a bag of the frozen forest fruits or summer berries instead. You can add the berries to the sponge mixture while they are still frozen.

1 Preheat oven to 180°C/350°F/gas mark 4. Grease a deep 20cm (8 inch) round or square cake tin.

2 Beat together the butter and sugar until soft and fluffy. Gradually add the eggs, beating well. You may need to add a little flour to stop the mixture from curdling.

3 Beat in the vanilla extract, then fold in the flour. Add the berries and gently stir to mix through.

4 Spoon the mixture into the prepared tin. Bake for 25-30 minutes, until golden on top and spongy to touch.

5 Leave to cool in the tin for a few minutes before transferring to a cooling rack. If freezing, leave to cool, wrap up in foil and freeze, or cut into slices and freeze individually.

6 To serve, defrost thoroughly, then mash or finely chop.

stewed plum crisp

makes: 4 portions

storage: up to 2-3 days in the refrigerator or up to 3 months in the freezer

400g (14oz) ripe plums, stoned and quartered
50g (1¾oz) light soft brown sugar, plus 1-2 tsp to taste
180g (6¼oz) wholemeal plain flour, plus 1 tbsp
¼ level tsp ground cinnamon, plus a pinch
110g (4oz) unsalted butter, cut into cubes and chilled

Try to use ripe plums that are naturally sweet so that you do not need to add much sugar. You could also try adding some oats to the crumble topping for extra fibre. Like all fruits, plums provide vitamins and minerals. If you want to mix the plums with another fruit, try adding sliced eating apples.

1 Preheat the oven to 180°C/350°F/gas mark 4.

2 Put the plums in a large bowl, add 1-2 tsp sugar to taste, 1 tbsp wholemeal flour, and a pinch of ground cinnamon.

3 Mix together gently and tip into a buttered ovenproof dish.

4 Sieve the 180g (6¼oz) flour and the ¼ level tsp of cinnamon into a bowl. Rub in the butter until the mixture looks like breadcrumbs. Stir in the 50g (1¾oz) of sugar. Sprinkle the crumble topping over the plums. If freezing, cool and then freeze.

5 Bake in the oven for 25 minutes, until bubbling and the top is golden. Finely chop.

tropical fruit fool

makes: approx. 6 portions

storage: best eaten immediately or up to 24 hours in the refrigerator

200ml (7fl oz) full-fat milk or soy drink
1 vanilla pod, split lengthways
3 free-range egg yolks
1 tsp caster sugar
1 tbsp cornflour
1 ripe mango
1 ripe passion fruit (or 1 ripe banana, chopped)
100g (3¾oz) natural full-fat yogurt

Goats' and sheeps' milk are both thought to be less likely to cause an allergic reaction than cows' milk, so they are a great way to introduce protein into your baby's diet – as part of a dish, rather than a drink. However, cows' milk, introduced very gradually in dishes, to babies at this age, is perfectly acceptable.

1 To make the custard, heat the milk with the vanilla pod in a saucepan until just below boiling point. Remove the vanilla pod at this point.

2 In a bowl, mix the egg yolks, sugar, and cornflour together. Pour the hot milk over this mixture, stirring constantly. Return to the saucepan and heat, stirring constantly, until the mixture thickens. Do not allow to boil, or it will curdle. Leave the custard to cool.

3 Meanwhile, cut the mango flesh either side of the stone, peel, and cut into chunks. Put into a bowl. Cut the passion fruit in half and scoop the pulp into the bowl. Alternatively, add the banana. Blend to a purée with a hand-held blender (or in a food processor or blender).

4 Gently fold together the cooled custard and yogurt. Swirl through the fruit purée to make a rippled fool.

apple flapjacks

makes: 15 baby portions

storage: 4–5 days in an airtight container, or up to 3 months in the freezer

125g (4½oz) unsalted butter
75g (2½oz) soft brown sugar
2 tbsp golden syrup
350g (12½oz) porridge oats
½ tsp baking powder
2 eating apples, peeled, cored and grated
50g (1¾oz) hazelnuts, toasted and ground

These are great flapjacks because they are soft, moist, and slightly crumbly, rather than hard and chewy, which can be too much for many babies. The apple gives a natural sweetness, so these flapjacks are not as sugar-laden as many store-bought ones. (Do not feed nuts to babies if there is any family history of allergies.)

1 Preheat the oven to 180°C/350°F/gas mark 4. Grease a 23cm x 33cm (9 inch x 13 inch) Swiss roll tin.

2 Melt the butter, sugar, and golden syrup together in a large saucepan over a low heat.

3 In a bowl, mix together the oats, baking powder, apples, and hazelnuts, stirring well. Add to the butter mixture and mix together.

4 Tip into the tin and flatten the surface. Bake for 20 minutes, until the edges are just beginning to turn golden. Cut into squares while still warm and leave to cool in the tin.

5 If freezing, layer with greaseproof paper and store in freezer bags. Freeze. Thaw thoroughly.

banana custard

makes: 10 baby portions

storage: 2 days in the refrigerator (without the banana added), or up to 3 months in the freezer

200ml (7fl oz) full-fat milk or calcium-enriched soy drink
1 vanilla pod, split lengthways
3 large free-range egg yolks
1 tsp golden caster sugar
1 tbsp cornflour
2 medium ripe bananas
100g (3¾oz) natural Greek yogurt

Bananas are a perennially popular food for babies, although you can try this recipe with mango instead of banana if you prefer.

1   To make the custard, heat the milk with the vanilla pod in a saucepan until just below boiling point. Remove from the heat and take out the vanilla pod.
2   In a bowl, mix the egg yolks, sugar, and cornflour together. Pour the hot milk over the egg mixture, stirring constantly until smooth.
3   Return to the saucepan and heat, stirring constantly, until the mixture thickens. Do not allow to boil or it will curdle.
4   Once the custard has thickened, leave it to cool.
5   Meanwhile, purée the bananas and yogurt together in a bowl with a hand-held blender (or in a food processor or blender). Gently fold together the cooled custard and banana mixture.
6   Spoon the purée into ice-cube trays. If freezing, cover with foil or put into a freezer bag and seal. Freeze for at least 4 hours, until frozen. Transfer to freezer bags and return to the freezer. Thaw thoroughly and heat gently until warm.

vanilla pears

makes: 3–4 baby portions, or 1 baby portion and 1 adult portion

storage: up to 24 hours in the refrigerator

2 ripe pears, such as Williams, peeled, cored and thinly sliced
1 tsp soft brown sugar
1 tbsp lemon juice
1 vanilla pod, sliced lengthways (optional)
small knob of unsalted butter
natural full-fat yogurt, to serve

This is a really delicious winter pudding, especially if you add a little pinch of ground ginger. If you have any left over, it's also very good cold served with yogurt or muesli for breakfast.

1   Preheat the oven to 180°C/350°F/gas mark 4.
2   Put the pears in an ovenproof dish, then toss them with the sugar, lemon juice, vanilla pod (if using), and butter.
3   Bake the pears for approximately 20 minutes, basting occasionally, until tender and golden.
4   To serve, remove the vanilla pod and finely chop or mash the pears. Serve with natural yogurt.

seasonal **foods**

	December	January	February	March	April	May
fruit						
apples	●	●	●	●	●	●
citrus fruits	●	●	●	●		
grapes	●	●				
pears	●	●	●			
rhubarb	●	●	●	●	●	●
beetroot	●	●	●			
vegetables						
broccoli				●	●	●
carrots		●	●	●	●	●
celery		●	●			
chard			●			
cucumbers				●	●	●
leeks				●	●	
mushrooms	●	●	●	●	●	●
onions	●	●	●			
parsnips	●	●	●			
potatoes (main)	●	●	●	●	●	●
potatoes (new)						●
spinach					●	●
sweet potatoes	●	●	●			

	June	July	August	September	October	November
fruit						
apples	●			●	●	●
apricots				●		
blackberries		●	●	●	●	
blueberries		●	●			
cherries	●	●	●			
peaches		●	●	●		
nectarines		●	●	●		
pears				●	●	●
plums			●			
rasberries	●	●	●	●	●	
rhubarb	●	●	●	●		●
strawberries	●	●	●	●	●	
vegetables						
asparagus	●					
aubergine				●	●	
beetroot	●	●	●	●	●	●
broad beans	●	●	●			
broccoli	●	●	●	●	●	●
carrots	●	●	●	●		
capiscum				●	●	
cucumbers	●	●	●	●	●	
mushrooms	●	●	●	●	●	●
peas	●	●	●			
potatoes (main)				●	●	●
potatoes (new)	●					
pumpkin			●	●	●	●
spinach	●	●	●	●	●	●
sweetcorn			●	●	●	
tomatoes		●	●	●		
watercress				●	●	●

organic
certificates

In the UK the government has created the UK Register of Organic Food Standards (UKROFS), which approves organic food inspection bodies (see table, right). These organisations ensure that farmers wishing to produce and sell organic products are thoroughly inspected and continue to maintain the high standards required. Once a farm has been approved, which means that a farmer has conformed to a set of guidelines on the production and processing of organic produce, it can label its produce with a certification symbol. Check the label to make sure that it carries one of these symbols.

The most widespread approved symbol in the UK is that of The Soil Association, which covers around 70-80 per cent of all certified organic food on sale in Britain.

The table (right) contains the various organic food inspection bodies that have been approved by the UK Register of Organic Food Standards. If organic products are imported, then EU regulations demand that they are inspected, approved and thus certified by one of these inspection bodies to the same standards as those applied in the UK and the rest of the EU.

Several worldwide bodies exist to regulate organic production and processing systems around the world so that what is considered organic in one country meets the standard of inspection in another.

guarantees and certification register

The Soil Association
Bristol House, 40-56 Victoria Street,
Bristol BS1 6BY
Tel: 0117 929 0661

Organic Farmers and Growers
Views Farm, Great Milton,
Oxford, Oxfordshire OX9 7NW
Tel: 01844 279352

DEMETER The Biodynamic Agricultural Association
Painswick Inn Project,
Gloucester Street, Stroud, Gloucestershire, GL5 1QG
Tel: 01453 759501

The Scottish Organic Producers Association
Milton of Cambus, Doone,
Perthshire FK16 6HG
Tel: 01786 841657

The Irish Organic Farmers and Growers Association
Harbour Building,
Harbour Road, Kilbeggan, County Westmeath,
Tel: 0506 32563

Organic Food Federation (OFF)
1 Mowles Manor, Enterprise Centre, Etling Green,
Dereham, Norfolk NR20 3EZ
Tel: 01362 637314

UKROFS (UK Register of Organic Food Standards), Ministry of Agriculture, Fisheries and Food
Noble House, 17 Smith Square, London SW1P 3JR Tel: 020 7238 5915

useful
addresses

The Vegetarian Society
Parkdale
Dunham Road
Altringham
Cheshire WA14 4QG
Tel: 0161 925 2000
www.vegsoc.org

Vegan Society
Donald Watson House
7 Battle Road
St. Leonards on Sea
East Sussex TN37 7AA
Tel: 01424 427393
www.vegansociety.com

La Leche League (Great Britain)
PO Box 29
West Bridgford
Nottingham NG2 7NP
Tel: 0845 456 1866 or 0115 981 5599
www.laleche.org.uk
Provide breastfeeding advice and support

National Childbirth Trust
Alexandra House
Oldham Terrace
Acton
London W3 6NH
Tel: 0870 770 3236
enquiries@national-childbirth-trust.co.uk
www.nat-online.org
*Provide support during pregnancy, childbirth,
and early parenthood*

Association of Breastfeeding Mothers
ABM PO Box 207
Bridgewater
Somerset TA6 7YT
Tel: 020 7813 1481
www.abm.me.uk

The Hyperactive Children's Support Group
71 Whyke Lane
Chichester
West Sussex PO19 7PD
Tel: 01903 725 182

Allergy UK
No.3 White Oak Square
London Road
Swanley
Kent BR8 7AG
Tel: 01322 619898
www.allergyuk.org

index